前　言

《循证针灸临床实践指南》包括：带状疱疹、贝尔面瘫、抑郁症、中风后假性球麻痹、偏头痛、颈椎病、慢性便秘、腰痛、原发性痛经、坐骨神经痛、失眠、成人支气管哮喘、肩周炎、膝关节炎、急慢性胃炎、过敏性鼻炎、突发性耳聋、三叉神经痛、糖尿病周围神经病变、单纯性肥胖病等病症的循证针灸临床实践指南。

本部分为《循证针灸临床实践指南》的慢性便秘部分。

本部分受国家中医药管理局指导与委托。

本部分由中国针灸学会提出。

本部分由中国针灸学会标准化工作委员会归口。

本部分起草单位：中国中医科学院广安门医院针灸科、中国中医科学院针灸研究所。

本部分主要起草人：张维、刘保延、刘志顺、张涛、彭唯娜。

本部分专家组成员：武晓冬、赵宏、房繁恭、吴泰相、吴中朝、杨金洪、梁繁荣、赵吉平、刘炜宏、杨金生、余曙光、郭义、杨骏、赵京生、詹思延、刘建平、杨华元、储浩然、石现、王富春、王麟鹏、贾春生、余晓阳、高希言、常小荣、张洪涛、吕明庄、王玲玲、宣丽华、翟伟、岗卫娟、王昕、董国锋、王芳。

引　言

《循证针灸临床实践指南》是根据针灸临床优势，针对特定临床情况，参照古代文献、名医经验以及现代最佳临床研究证据，结合患者价值观和意愿，系统研制的帮助临床医生和患者做出恰当针灸处理的指导性意见。

《循证针灸临床实践指南》制定的总体思路是：在针灸实践与临床研究的基础上，遵循循证医学的理念与方法，紧紧围绕针灸临床的特色优势，综合专家经验、目前最佳证据以及患者价值观，将国际公认的证据质量评价与推荐方案分级的规范与古代、前人、名老针灸专家临床证据相结合，并将临床研究证据与大范围专家共识相结合，旨在制定出能保障针灸临床疗效和安全性、并具有科学性与实用性的可有效指导针灸临床实践的指导性意见。

在《循证针灸临床实践指南》的制定过程中，各专家组共同参与，还完成了国家标准《针灸临床实践指南制定与评估规范》（以下简称《规范》）的送审稿。《规范》参照了国际上临床实践指南制定的要求和经验，根据中国国情以及针灸的发展状况，对《循证针灸临床实践指南》制定的组织、人员、过程、采用证据质量评价、推荐方案等级划分、专家共识形成方式、制定与更新的内容和时间等都进行了规范。这些规范性要求在《循证针灸临床实践指南》制定中都得到了充分考量与完善。《规范》与《循证针灸临床实践指南》相辅相成，《规范》是《循证针灸临床实践指南》制定的指导，《循证针灸临床实践指南》又是《规范》适用性的验证实例。

《循证针灸临床实践指南》推荐等级主要采用世界卫生组织（WHO）等推荐的 GRADE（Grading of Recommendations Assessment，Development and Evaluation）系统，即推荐分级的评价、制定与评估的系统，其中推荐等级分为强推荐与弱推荐两级。强推荐的方案是估计变化可能性较小，个性化程度低的方案，而弱推荐方案则是估计变化可能性较大，个性化程度高，患者价值观差异大的方案。对于古代文献和名医经验的证据质量评价，目前课题组还在进一步研制中，《循证针灸临床实践指南》仅将古代文献和名医经验作为证据之一附列在现代证据后面，供《循证针灸临床实践指南》使用者参考。

2008 年，在 WHO 西太区的项目资助下，由中国中医科学院牵头、中国针灸学会标准化工作委员会组织完成了针灸治疗带状疱疹、贝尔面瘫、抑郁症、中风后假性球麻痹和偏头痛 5 种病症的指南研制工作。在这 5 种病症的指南研制过程中，课题组初步提出了《循证针灸临床实践指南》的研究方法和建议，建立了《循证针灸临床实践指南》的体例、研究模式与技术路线。2010 年 12 月，《临床病症中医临床实践指南·针灸分册》由中国中医药出版社正式出版发行。

2009 年至 2013 年，在国家中医药管理局立项支持下，中国针灸学会标准化工作委员会又先后分 3 批启动了 15 种病症的指南研制工作。为了保证《循证针灸临床实践指南》高质量地完成，在总课题组的组织下，由四川大学华西医院吴泰相教授在京举办 2 次 GRADE 方法学培训会议，全国 11 家临床及科研单位的 100 多位学员接受了培训。随后，总课题组又组织了 15 个疾病临床指南制定课题组和 1 个方法学课题组中的 17 位研究人员，赴华西医院循证医学中心接受了为期 3 个月的 Meta 分析和 GRADE 方法学专题培训，受训研究人员系统学习并掌握了 GRADE 系统证据质量评价和推荐意见形成的方法。

本次出版的《循证针灸临床实践指南》共有 20 个部分，包括对 2010 年版 5 部分指南的修订再版和 2013 年完成的 15 部分指南的首次出版。《循证针灸临床实践指南》的适用对象为从事针灸临床与科研的专业人员。

《循证针灸临床实践指南》的证据质量分级和推荐强度等级如下：

◇证据质量分级

证据质量高：A

证据质量中：B

证据质量低：C

证据质量极低：D

◇推荐强度等级

支持使用某项干预措施的强推荐：1

支持使用某项干预措施的弱推荐：2

《循证针灸临床实践指南》的编写，凝聚着全国针灸标准化科研人员和管理人员的辛勤汗水，是参与研制各方集体智慧的结晶，是辨证论治的个体化诊疗模式与循证医学有机结合的创造性探索。《循证针灸临床实践指南》在研制过程中，得到了兰州大学循证医学中心杨克虎教授、陈耀龙博士以及北京大学循证医学中心詹思延教授在方法学上的大力支持和帮助，在此深表感谢。同时，还要感谢国家中医药管理局政策法规与监督司领导的热心指导与大力支持；此外，还要感谢各位专家的通力合作；在《循证针灸临床实践指南》的出版过程中，中国中医药出版社表现出了很高的专业水平，在此一并致谢。

摘　　要

1　治疗原则

针灸治疗慢性便秘应在明确病理分型及病因的基础上，以对症处理为主，总体原则为通腑导滞；取穴应体现"气至病所"的特点，以腹部穴位为主，直接刺激病变部位；亦可通过经络理论指导下的远端取穴间接刺激病变部位；取穴数目通常较少，可考虑使用单穴治疗。

2　主要推荐意见

	推荐意见		推荐级别
慢性功能性便秘（未明确分型）	方案1：对于未进行病理分型的慢性功能性便秘患者，推荐采用深刺天枢穴加电针疗法治疗		强推荐
	方案2：对于不能或不愿接受针刺治疗的慢性功能性便秘患者，推荐采用耳穴压丸疗法治疗		弱推荐
结肠慢传输型便秘	方案1：推荐采用深刺天枢穴加电针疗法治疗		强推荐
	方案2：对于不能或不愿接受针刺治疗的患者，推荐采用热敏灸法治疗		弱推荐
慢性功能性便秘（肠道气滞型）	推荐采用电针支沟穴治疗		弱推荐
老年慢性功能性便秘	推荐以"靳三针"中的肠三针、四神针、脑三针、足三针配合治疗		强推荐
便秘型肠易激综合征	在具备人员和门诊手术条件的医疗单位，在充分考虑患者意愿的前提下，推荐采用指针配合穴位埋线疗法治疗		弱推荐
盆底失弛缓综合征	方案1：推荐以毫针刺法结合生物反馈治疗		弱推荐
	方案2：推荐以深刺中髎、下髎穴治疗		弱推荐
糖尿病性便秘	推荐以毫针刺法结合中药疗法治疗		弱推荐

简　　介

《循证针灸临床实践指南：慢性便秘》（以下简称《指南》）简介如下：

1　本《指南》制定的目标

本《指南》制定的目标是为临床医生推荐证据可靠的慢性便秘的针灸诊疗方案，提高临床疗效。

2　本《指南》制定的目的

本《指南》制定的目的是确定慢性便秘的针灸诊治策略、针灸治疗建议、推荐方案、操作规范及注意事项等。

3　本《指南》的适用人群

本《指南》的适用人群主要为国内针灸从业者、中医药院校的教师和学生、从事针灸专业的科研工作者等。

4　本《指南》适用的疾病范围

本《指南》适用的疾病范围包括所有符合各专业学术组织所制定诊断标准的慢性功能性便秘，以及部分由患者基础疾病导致的器质性便秘。

概　述

1　定义

1.1　西医

便秘是由多种病因引起的一种病症，以排便次数减少（1周内大便次数少于2~3次或2~3天才大便1次）、粪便量减少、粪便干结、排出困难为主要表现，部分患者可合并一些特殊症状（如长时间用力排便，直肠胀感，排便不尽感，甚至需用手法帮助排便），病程至少6个月以上者，属慢性便秘[1-2]。

1.2　中医

便秘是指粪便在肠内滞留过久，秘结不通，排便周期延长，或周期不长，但粪质干结，排出艰难，或粪质不硬，虽有便意，但排便不畅的病证。便秘多因大肠积热、气滞、寒凝或气血阴阳亏虚而使肠道传导功能失常所致。《内经》称便秘为"大便难""后不利"，古代相关文献载有"脾约""闭""阳结""阴结""大便秘""大便燥结""便闭""肠结""风秘""气秘""虚秘""热秘""三焦秘""幽门秘""直肠结""湿秘""热燥""风燥"等十余种名称。

2　发病率及人群分布情况

流行病学资料显示，我国各地的便秘患病率有很大差异，在3%~17%之间，并随年龄的增长，便秘的患病率明显增加[3]。儿童患病率约为3.8%[4]。随着饮食结构的改变和精神心理、社会因素的影响，我国慢性便秘的患病率逐渐上升。北京地区18~70岁人群进行的随机、分层调查表明，慢性便秘的患病率为6.07%[5]，年龄增长则便秘的患病率明显增加[6]，女性患病率略高于男性，农村人口的患病率高于城市人口。便秘的发生与紧张、疲劳等精神心理因素、生活方式、饮食习惯及便秘家族史有关[7]，高脂饮食、吸烟史、低体重指数、文化程度低者更易发生便秘[8]。

临床特点

1 分类[1]

便秘依据病因的不同，可分为器质性便秘与功能性便秘两类。器质性便秘可由胃肠道疾病、累及消化道的系统性疾病（如糖尿病、硬皮病、神经系统疾病等）引起，许多药物也可引起便秘；而功能性便秘则不存在以上病因。

根据临床表现和病理特点的不同，便秘又可分为慢传输型、出口梗阻型和混合型三个类型。值得说明的是，以上分类方法既适合于功能性便秘，也适合于其他病因引起的器质性便秘。例如，糖尿病合并的便秘以及药物引起的便秘多是慢传输型便秘。便秘型肠易激综合征的特点是排便次数少，排便艰难，排便、排气后腹痛或腹胀缓解或减轻，多属于出口梗阻型合并慢传输型便秘。

根据症状的严重程度，可将便秘分为轻、中、重三度。轻度指症状较轻，不影响生活，经一般处理能好转，无需用药或少量用药即可解决。重度指便秘症状持续，患者异常痛苦，严重影响生活，不能停药或多次治疗无效。中度则鉴于两者之间。

2 症状及体征

临床上便秘常表现为便意少、便次减少（粪便不一定干硬）；排便艰难、费力（突出表现为粪便排出异常艰难）；排便不畅（有肛门直肠内阻塞感，虽频有便意，便次不少，但即使费力也无济于事，难有通畅的排便）；便秘常伴有腹痛或腹部不适，并常于排便后症状缓解。

3 临床检查

3.1 一般检查方法

临床上对于便秘患者，血常规、便常规、大便潜血试验和直肠指检是常规检查的内容。必要时可进行有关生化和代谢方面的检查及 X 线检查。对可疑肛门、直肠病变者，可选用直肠镜或乙状结肠镜、结肠镜检查，或钡剂灌肠等。

3.2 特殊检查方法

特殊检查包括胃肠通过试验（gastro－intestinal transit test，GITT）、肛门直肠测压（ano－rectal manometry，ARM）、结肠压力监测、气囊排出试验（balloon expulsion test，BET）、排粪造影（barium defecography，BD）、会阴神经潜伏期或肌电图检查等。对伴有明显焦虑和抑郁的患者，应做有关的调查，并判断其和便秘的因果关系。以上检查能够科学评估肠道与肛门直肠的功能，对便秘的分型、治疗以及疗效的评估具有重要意义[9]。

3.3 诊疗流程

根据 2005 年中华消化学会胃肠动力学组发布的《我国慢性便秘的诊治指南》，临床上为了做到对便秘患者进行有效的分层（报警与否）、分级（程度）、分流诊治，需要评估引起便秘的病因和诱因、便秘的类型以及程度。对有报警征象（如便血、贫血、消瘦、发热、黑便、腹痛等），或怀疑有器质性疾病引起的便秘时，应进一步检查，除外或证实有无器质性疾病，尤其是结肠肿瘤；对确定是器质性疾病的便秘患者，除了病因治疗外，同时也需要根据便秘的特点，判断便秘的类型，进行相应的治疗；对经验治疗或经检查未证实是器质性便秘的病例，进一步检查可以确定便秘的类型，再进行相应的治疗；对少数难治性便秘患者，一开始就进行有关的便秘类型检查，甚至更详细的检查，以便确定治疗手段。针灸临床也应严格按照诊疗流程进行必要的检查与鉴别。

诊断标准

1 西医诊断标准

2006 年 11 月，国际 Rome 协作委员会在 RomeⅡ的基础上，制定了 RomeⅢ功能性胃肠疾病的一系列诊断标准[9]。以下介绍有关 RomeⅢ的功能性便秘、盆底排便障碍及便秘型肠易激综合征的诊断标准。

1.1 功能性便秘诊断标准[10]

诊断前症状出现至少 6 个月，近 3 个月满足以下标准。

必须满足以下 2 条或多条：①排便费力（至少每 4 次排便中有 1 次）；②排便为块状或硬便（至少每 4 次排便中有 1 次）；③有排便不尽感（至少每 4 次排便中有 1 次）；④有肛门直肠梗阻和/或阻塞感（至少每 4 次排便中有 1 次）；⑤需要用手操作（如手指辅助排便、盆底支撑排便）以促进排便（至少每 4 次排便中有 1 次）；⑥排便少于每周 3 次。

不用缓泻药几乎没有松散大便。

诊断为肠易激综合征的条件不充分。

1.2 盆底排便障碍诊断标准[10]

除了符合功能性便秘的诊断标准之外，还需符合以下几点：①必须要有肛门直肠测压、肌电图或 X 线检查的证据，表明在反复做排便动作时，盆底肌群出现不合适的收缩或不能放松；②用力排便时，直肠能出现足够的推进性收缩；③有粪便排出不畅的证据。

1.3 便秘型肠易激综合征（便秘型 IBS）诊断标准

首先符合肠易激综合征诊断标准的基本点[10]，即在过去 12 个月内至少存在 12 周（不一定连续）有腹痛或腹部不适的症状，伴以下 3 条中的 2 条者：①便后上诉症状消失；②上述症状出现，同时伴有大便次数的改变；③伴有大便性状的改变。

同时，有以下 3 项表现中任何 1 项的支持：①便次少于 3 次/周；②稀便；③排便紧迫感。

2 中医诊断标准及分型

根据中华中医药学会脾胃病分会制定的慢性便秘中医诊疗共识意见 2011（北京）[11]，将便秘分为以下 5 型。证候确定标准：主症必备，加次症 2 项以上即可诊断。

2.1 肠道实热证

主症：大便干结，舌红，苔黄燥。

次症：腹中胀满或痛，口干口臭，心烦不寐，小便短赤，脉滑数。

2.2 肠道气滞证

主症：欲便不得出，或便而不爽，大便干结或不干，腹满胀痛。

次症：肠鸣矢气，嗳气频作，烦躁易怒或郁郁寡欢，纳食减少，舌苔薄腻，脉弦。

2.3 肺脾气虚证

主症：大便并不干硬，虽有便意，但排便困难，用力努挣则汗出短气。

次症：便后乏力，神疲懒言，舌淡苔白，脉弱。

2.4 脾肾阳虚证

主症：大便干或不干，排出困难，脉沉迟。

次症：腹中冷痛，得热则减，小便清长，四肢不温，面色㿠白，舌淡苔白。

2.5 津亏血少证

主症：大便干结，便如羊粪，舌红少苔或舌淡苔白。

次症：口干少津，眩晕耳鸣，腰膝酸软，心悸怔忡，两颧红赤，脉弱。

治疗概况

1 现代文献

针对便秘患者可进行包括调整饮食、适当运动、心理疗法和排便指导在内的一般性治疗。

药物治疗主要分为泻剂、促胃肠动力药、微生态制剂、灌肠剂和栓剂等。其中，泻剂又可分为容积性泻剂、渗透性泻剂、刺激性泻剂、润滑性泻剂和盐类泻剂5种[12-14]。渗透性泻剂中的聚乙二醇和乳果糖被列为A类证据[15-17]，其他药物的循证医学证据尚不充分。刺激性泻剂长期应用可引起水样腹泻、腹痛、水和电解质紊乱、变态反应、肝毒性反应及结肠黑变病等[18]，临床应用应谨慎。促胃肠动力药包括胃复安、吗丁啉、西沙必利、莫沙必利、普卡比利、替加色罗等。因西沙比利与替加色罗在心血管方面的不良反应，现已停用。

另外，还可选用非药物治疗，包括大肠水疗法、生物反馈疗法、神经肌肉刺激疗法、胃肠起搏疗法和电子药丸等[19-27]。

对于经药物长期治疗无效的慢性顽固性便秘患者，可在严格评价后行外科手术治疗。近年来，研究发现手术无效率和复发率均较高，不能作为便秘的常规治疗手段，故对于慢性便秘的治疗，更多地恢复到以非手术治疗为主，对手术适应证的限制也越来越严[34]。

2 古代文献

便秘在《内经》中称为"大便难""后不利"，其他古代相关文献中载有"脾约""大便不利""大便燥结"等十余种名称。古代医家针灸治疗便秘的特点是：辨证治疗以脾为主，多选肾经、膀胱经、脾经的穴位，以远端取穴为主，多行浅刺，重用灸法。

3 名医经验

针灸治疗本病的方法多种多样，临床研究均报道了其较高的临床疗效和较好的安全性，已经成为便秘临床干预很有前景和潜力的方法。

目前临床治疗便秘最常用的针刺方法有毫针刺法、芒针刺法、头针刺法、电针疗法、穴位埋线疗法、穴位注射疗法、耳针疗法（包括耳穴压丸疗法）、皮内埋针疗法等。多种针刺方法虽各具特点，但目的都是"气至病所"，起到导滞通便的作用。

现代名医治疗慢性便秘，常用的配穴方案一般有单穴治疗、特定穴组治疗以及辨证取穴3种。单穴应用最多的穴位是天枢、大肠俞、上巨虚、足三里等。常用的特定穴组有合募配穴、募俞配穴等。根据脏腑、经络、气血津液辨证取穴，能更全面地综合病情，对证施治。另外，知名针灸专家经验穴治疗也取得不错的疗效，如肠胃积热者配合谷、曲池、支沟、内庭；气机瘀滞者配中脘、阳陵泉、行间、支沟、太冲、大敦等。国内有研究者应用特定针刺手法（如烧山火等）治疗功能性便秘，具有一定的疗效。

根据现有的临床研究结果，针灸疗法对于某些类型的便秘，如结肠慢传输型便秘、便秘型肠易激综合征等有良好的治疗效果[28-30]。

针灸治疗和推荐方案

1 针灸治疗的原则及特点

1.1 治疗总则

便秘可以是某些疾病的症状之一，也可以单独作为一种疾病存在。临床凡见大便排出困难，排便次数减少，且病程超过半年者，均可纳入慢性便秘的范畴。针灸治疗便秘，应在明确病理分型及病因的基础上，以对症处理为主，总体原则为通腑导滞。

1.2 选穴处方特点

慢性便秘的针灸选穴充分体现了"气至病所"的特点，以腹部穴位为主，直接刺激病变部位；亦可通过经络理论指导下的远端取穴间接刺激病变部位；背俞穴具有内合脏腑的特点，可以调节肠腑的功能，缓解便秘的症状，可考虑选用；取穴数目较少，可考虑使用单穴治疗。

1.2.1 腹部穴位为主

便秘为肠腑受病，由大肠积热、气滞、寒凝或气血阴阳亏虚，使得肠道传导功能失常所致，所以针刺腹部穴位治疗便秘机理明确，作用直接，每获良效。

1.2.2 远端取穴

远端肢体取穴在古代文献中即有记述，《杂病穴法歌》曰："大便虚秘补支沟，泻足三里效可拟。"某些远端穴位，如支沟穴可通畅三焦，达到行气通便的作用。

1.2.3 背俞穴

背俞穴是脏腑经气汇聚于背部的穴位，对背俞穴进行针灸刺激，可通过经络系统等内在途径调节肠腑的功能，通利大便。

1.2.4 取穴精简，可用单穴

根据临床研究报道，对于某些类型的便秘，取单穴针刺即可获得良效，为操作简便起见，一般不建议取穴过多。

1.3 针灸治疗的特点

1.3.1 针刺深度是影响临床疗效的关键

在"腹深如井"的理论支持下，腹部穴位可适度深刺，但必须掌握个体化原则，"中病即止"，并严格按照相关规定进行操作。

1.3.2 电针疗法在慢性便秘的针灸治疗中使用较为普遍

在针刺腹部穴位的过程中，多数研究采用电针作为刺激方式，可加强肠道蠕动，增进疗效。

1.3.3 疗程及疗程间隔

慢性便秘针灸治疗建议每周3次，周六、日休息，2周为1个疗程，疗程间隔2天。根据便秘的严重程度调整治疗次数，重度便秘患者可每周治疗5次。同时，对于治疗后效果不佳的便秘患者，允许在针灸疗程内随时采取其他通便措施或至专科诊治。

2 主要结局指标

依据 GRADE 证据质量评价系统，结局指标的重要程度分为 1~9 共9个等级，其中 1~3 为 Not Important（对决策影响不大的结果），4~6 为 Important（影响决策的重要而非关键结果），7~9 为 Critical（影响决策的关键结果）。每级又分为三个数值，数值越大，重要性越大。据统计，所有针灸治疗慢性便秘的文献共涉及结局评价指标21个，根据以上原则，结合慢性便秘的临床研究特点，拟定结局指标的重要程度分级为：9：患者对治疗的满意度；8：暂缺；7：治疗有效（痊愈）率；6：结肠运转时间（CTT）；5：生活质量评分（PAC – QOL）；4：心理症状自评量表（SCL – 90）；3：包

括 CCS 评分、大便形状，治疗后首次自主排便距治疗结束时间，自主排便次数差，治疗前后排便时间差异，治疗前后及治疗中症状总积分差，治疗前后 72 小时结肠标志物排出率差值比较，治疗前后粪便性状正常率，抑郁自评量表 SDS，焦虑自评量表 SAS，治疗前后排便速度差，治疗前后大便性状差，治疗前后排便难度积分差，治疗前后便意积分差，治疗前后排便间隔时间差，排便不尽感差值，排便频率评分差值，共 16 项。建议不要使用自拟的标准进行疗效评价。

3 注意事项

3.1 消毒方法

采用 75% 酒精或安尔碘进行针刺部位的常规消毒。

3.2 操作要点

针刺腹部穴位须严格按照《针法灸法学》的相关规定，缓慢直刺，不做大幅度提插手法。

腹部穴位的针刺深度以患者获得针感为度，不建议过度深刺。

针刺后 3 天仍未排便的患者，建议采用其他通便措施或至专科诊治。

4 患者自我护理

针刺后 1 天内不要淋浴，不要污染针孔。

饮食宜清淡，可适当增加高纤维食物的摄入。

保证适量的户外活动。

5 推荐方案

5.1 慢性功能性便秘

2006 年 11 月，国际 Rome 协作委员会在 Rome Ⅱ 的基础上，制定了 Rome Ⅲ 慢性功能性便秘的诊断标准。根据病理特点的不同，慢性功能性便秘尚可进一步分为慢传输型、出口梗阻型和混合型三个类型。同时，慢性功能性便秘的病情严重程度及治疗效果受到诸多因素的影响，中医辨证分型、年龄等因素在确定患者治疗方案的过程中均应予以考虑。

5.1.1 未明确分型的慢性功能性便秘

由于受到临床检查条件及研究者对便秘分型的认识等方面的局限，诸多临床研究仅在符合 Rome Ⅲ 功能性便秘诊断标准的基础上纳入患者进行研究，并未针对便秘进一步分型。此类临床证据虽然在临床分型方面尚欠详细，但因其涵盖了临床针灸治疗便秘的大部分患者群体，指导意义较强。

方案一：深刺天枢穴加电针疗法

天枢穴为大肠经之募穴，腑气之所通。深刺法当属《灵枢·官针》中"输刺"的范畴，"输刺者，直出直入，稀发针而深之，以治气盛而热者也。"所以，在保证安全的前提下，可以考虑深刺此穴，以达到最佳的疗效。

取穴：天枢（双侧）。

针刺方法：采用直径 0.38mm、长度 75mm 的毫针快速破皮，然后缓慢垂直深刺，直至突破腹膜即止，不提插捻转，再连接电针仪电极于双侧针柄上。电针参数：等幅 2/15Hz。电流强度以患者腹部肌肉轻度颤动并自觉微痛为度。留针 30 分钟。突破腹膜的标准：操作者有破空感，同时病人有明显的揪痛感。

疗程：每日 1 次，每周治疗 5 次，连续治疗 4 周。疗程间休息 2 天，可治疗 2~3 个疗程。

注意事项：①腹主动脉瘤、肝脾异常肿大、肠麻痹、不全肠梗阻和腹腔结核者，不可使用本法。②安装心脏起搏器者，不可使用电针。

『推荐』

推荐建议：对于未进行病理分型的慢性功能性便秘患者，推荐采用深刺天枢穴加电针疗法治疗。[GRADE 1B]

解释：本《指南》小组共纳入相关文献 3 篇[31-33]，经综合分析，形成证据体发现，深刺天枢穴加电针治疗未分型的慢性功能性便秘，可有效改善患者结肠转运时间及自觉症状。但纳入的文献偏倚风险较高，证据体质量等级经 GRADE 评价后，因其纳入文献不精确性，最终证据体质量等级为中。

方案二：耳穴压丸疗法

耳穴压丸疗法是通过刺激人体各个部位在耳郭上的反应点或反射区来改善便秘。耳穴压丸疗效持久、节省时间、操作方便、痛苦小、经济安全，对于条件所限、无法规律接受针刺治疗者，或体弱、合并心血管疾患、无法承受针刺刺激量的患者群体较为适用。

取穴：①主穴：直肠下段、大肠、交感、便秘点。②配穴：三焦、肺、小肠。

操作方法：将表面光滑近以圆球状或椭圆状的王不留行籽，贴于 0.6cm×0.6cm 的小块胶布中央，然后对准耳穴贴紧并稍加压力，使患者耳朵感到酸、麻、胀或发热。贴后嘱患者每天自行按压数次，每次 1~2 分钟。

疗程：每次贴压后保持 3~7 天。3~6 次为 1 个疗程。

注意事项：①耳郭局部如存在破溃感染情况则不适合使用本法。②治疗过程中，贴压部位应保持干燥。

『推荐』

> 推荐建议：对于不能或不愿接受针刺治疗的慢性功能性便秘患者，推荐采用耳穴压丸疗法治疗。[GRADE 2D]

解释：本《指南》小组共纳入相关文献 5 篇[34-38]，经综合分析，形成证据体发现，耳穴压丸疗法可改善未明确分型的慢性功能性便秘患者 CCS 评分等。但纳入的文献偏倚风险较高，证据体质量等级经 GRADE 评价后，因其纳入文献设计质量低、证据间接及不精确性，最终证据体质量等级为极低。

5.1.2 结肠慢传输型便秘

结肠慢传输型便秘属于慢性功能性便秘的其中一种类型，该型患者结肠转运时间显著延长，因此结肠转运时间测定是诊断本病的特异性指标，临床有一定的发病率，治疗较为困难。近年来，针灸治疗结肠慢传输型便秘的临床研究逐渐增多，一定数量的临床证据表明，针灸对于结肠慢传输型便秘有相对确切的治疗作用。

方案一：深刺天枢穴加电针疗法

深刺天枢穴加电针对于结肠慢传输型便秘同样表现出较为显著的治疗效果。

其针刺方法、疗程及注意事项可参见 5.1.1 的相关内容。

『推荐』

> 推荐建议：推荐采用深刺天枢穴加电针疗法治疗结肠慢传输型便秘。[GRADE 1B]

解释：本《指南》小组共纳入相关文献 4 篇[39-42]，经综合分析，形成证据体发现，深刺天枢穴加电针治疗结肠慢传输性便秘，可有效改善患者结肠转运时间及 CCS 评分。但纳入的文献偏倚风险较高，证据体质量等级经 GRADE 评价后，因其纳入文献不一致性及不精确性，最终证据体质量等级为中。

方案二：热敏灸法

热敏灸法是近年来出现的一种新型灸法。人体在病理状态下，体表可产生一种反应（即腧穴热敏化现象），表现为对艾条温热刺激的敏感，这种现象称为腧穴热敏化现象。发生热敏化现象的部位称为热敏点或热敏化腧穴，在热敏点上施灸以治疗相关疾病的方法即为热敏灸法。由于灸法是非侵入性疗法，与针刺治疗相比，操作简便，对于不能或不愿接受针刺治疗的患者可予以采用。

取穴：在慢性便秘的热敏化高发区寻找热敏点（背部足太阳膀胱经左右两条第二侧线以内，肾俞和大肠俞两穴水平线之间的区域范围内）。

操作方法：在探查到的每个热敏点中，分别依次按照回旋灸、雀啄灸、往返灸、温和灸四步进行灸法操作。具体步骤是：先行回旋灸 2 分钟，温热局部气血；继行雀啄灸 1 分钟，加强敏化；再行循经往返灸 2 分钟，激发经气；最后行温和灸发动感传，开通经络。施行温和灸直至热敏现象消失为一次施灸剂量。完成一次治疗的施灸时间因人而异，一般为 10～120 分钟不等，施灸时间以热敏点的热敏现象消失为度。

疗程：隔日 1 次，4 周为 1 个疗程。

注意事项：施灸过程中，注意热度调节，如患者感觉疼痛则需要及时调整艾条与皮肤的距离，避免烫伤。

『推荐』

> 推荐建议：对于不能或不愿接受针刺治疗的患者，推荐采用热敏灸法治疗结肠慢传输型便秘。[GRADE 2D]

解释：本《指南》小组共纳入相关文献 1 篇[43]，经综合分析，形成证据体发现，热敏灸法可有效缓解大便排出困难，改善大便性状。但纳入的文献偏倚风险较高，证据体质量等级经 GRADE 评价后，因其纳入文献设计质量低及不精确性，最终证据体质量等级为极低。

5.1.3 参考中医辨证分型的慢性功能性便秘（肠道气滞型便秘）

针灸治疗是中医学的一部分，因此，在依据 RomeⅢ标准确定诊断的基础上进行中医辨证分型是必要的，较为有限的临床证据支持针灸辨证分型治疗慢性功能性便秘。这里重点介绍肠道气滞型慢性便秘的针灸治疗。

五脏气机的调畅，是大肠正常传导的基础，气机不通则每见排便费力、艰涩不畅、胸胁痞满、腹中胀痛、嗳气频作等症。三焦气机畅达则腑气通畅，故治便秘可考虑以"调气通腑"为原则，取三焦经的穴位针刺以调理三焦气机，畅达下焦，通利大便。

方案：针刺支沟穴

取穴：支沟穴（双侧）。

针刺方法：穴位处常规皮肤消毒，取直径 0.35mm、长度 50mm 的毫针垂直刺入，针刺深度以得气为度，行平补平泻法 30 秒，留针 30 分钟。

疗程：每日 1 次，7 天为 1 个疗程，可连续治疗 4 个疗程。

注意事项：针刺过程中，如患者感觉针刺部位有串电样针感并向手指尖放射，则应将针具提至皮下部位，改变方向再行针刺，避免损伤正中神经。

『推荐』

> 推荐建议：推荐针刺支沟穴治疗肠道气滞型慢性便秘。[GRADE 2C]

解释：本《指南》小组共纳入相关文献 1 篇[44]，经综合分析，形成证据体发现，针刺支沟穴治疗肠道气滞型便秘，可明显减轻排便不尽感，改善大便性状。但纳入的文献偏倚风险较高，证据体质量等级经 GRADE 评价后，因其纳入文献设计质量低、证据间接及不精确性，最终证据体质量等级为低。

5.1.4 老年慢性功能性便秘

临床流行病学研究已经证实，随着年龄的增长，便秘的患病率明显增加。人到老年，五脏虚衰，阴阳气血俱虚，治疗难度较大，且心理因素对于病情及治疗效果有一定的影响。所以，老年慢性功能性便秘的针灸治疗需要兼顾诸多方面，共同起到调神、理气、通腑的作用。

方案："靳三针"疗法

取穴：①肠三针：天枢（双侧）、关元、上巨虚（双侧）。②四神针：百会穴前后左右各 1.5 寸。③脑三针：脑户穴和左右脑空穴共 3 穴。④足三针：足三里（双侧）、三阴交（双侧）、太冲（双侧）。

针刺方法：腹部和肢体穴位选用直径 0.38mm、长度 40mm 的毫针，进针 1 ~ 1.5 寸。肠三针、足三里、三阴交用捻转补法，余穴用平补平泻法。

捻转手法操作：用拇指和食指持针，通过拇指、食指来回旋转捻动。捻转时，拇指与食指用力均匀，捻转幅度小，拇指向前左转时用力重，拇指向后右转还原时用力轻，反复操作。留针 30 分钟，每 10 分钟行针 1 次。

疗程：每日 1 次，4 次为 1 个疗程，疗程间休息 3 天，依病情治疗 1 ~ 3 个疗程。

注意事项：行捻转手法时，应注意保持捻转频率均匀一致，避免过度用力及单向捻转，防止出现滞针等情况。

『推荐』

> 推荐建议：推荐以"靳三针"中的肠三针、四神针、脑三针、足三针配合治疗老年慢性功能性便秘。[GRADE 1C]

解释：本《指南》小组共纳入相关文献 1 篇[45]，经综合分析，形成证据体发现，"靳三针"疗法治疗老年慢性便秘可改善结肠通过时间，提高粪便性状正常率。但纳入的文献偏倚风险较高，证据体质量等级经 GRADE 评价后，因其纳入文献证据间接及不精确性，最终证据体质量等级为低。

5.2 便秘型肠易激综合征

肠易激综合征是一种常见的功能性肠道疾病，主要分为便秘型、腹痛型和腹泻型。Rome 协作委员会同样在 RomeⅢ 当中制定了便秘型肠易激综合征的诊断标准。

方案：指针配合穴位埋线疗法

取穴：大肠俞（双侧）、肺俞（双侧）、肝俞（双侧）、天枢（双侧）、足三里（双侧）、上巨虚（双侧）、关元、中脘。

操作方法：①指针治疗：嘱患者双手抱枕俯卧于治疗床上，操作者沿患者双侧足太阳膀胱经第一侧线自上而下，先后施予按揉法、扪法及捏法。每次操作 15 分钟，每日 1 次，连续治疗 7 天。②穴位埋线治疗：指针治疗 10 天后，继予穴位埋线治疗。常规消毒穴位皮肤，取 3 号医用羊肠线，用注线法将羊肠线埋在穴位皮下组织或肌层内，埋入后针孔用碘伏消毒，敷盖无菌敷料。

疗程：每周穴位埋线 1 次，4 周为 1 个疗程。

注意事项：①严格执行无菌操作，建议在有门诊手术条件的医疗单位完成。②施术者在进行埋线治疗前应进行必要的培训，以熟练掌握操作要点。③治疗后 3 天之内，每日用碘伏消毒针眼 1 次，预防感染。

『推荐』

> 推荐建议：在具备人员和门诊手术条件的医疗单位，在充分考虑患者意愿的前提下，推荐采用指针配合穴位埋线疗法治疗便秘型肠易激综合征。[GRADE 2D]

解释：本《指南》小组共纳入相关文献 1 篇[46]，经综合分析，形成证据体发现，指针配合穴位埋线疗法治疗便秘型肠易激综合征，可有效改善结肠通过时间，改善大便性状。但纳入的文献偏倚风险较高，证据体质量等级经 GRADE 评价后，因其纳入文献设计质量低及不精确性，最终证据体质量等级为极低。

5.3 盆底失弛缓综合征

盆底失弛缓综合征是盆底肌反射性或随意性异常而引起的一组症候群，其临床特征是排便时盆底肌不松弛，反而异常收缩，阻塞盆底出口，引起排便困难。多数研究者认为，盆底失弛缓综合征是出口梗阻型便秘的一种。1995年，上海长海医院李实忠教授首先提出了"盆底失弛缓综合征"这一名称，较为直接准确地揭示了该病的病理本质，被业界广为接受。

方案一：毫针刺法结合生物反馈疗法

取穴：第1组取天枢、气海、上巨虚、足三里、百会；第2组取中髎、下髎、大肠俞、肾俞、脾俞、神道。

操作方法：①针灸治疗：a. 两组穴位轮流交替使用。b. 天枢、大肠俞直刺2~2.5寸，得气后施平补平泻法；气海、肾俞直刺1.5寸，脾俞直刺0.5寸，得气后施补法；上巨虚、足三里直刺1~1.5寸，得气后施平补平泻法；中髎、下髎刺入3寸（针入骶后孔2.5寸），强刺激，使针感放射至肛门。c. 百会、神道用低频率、小角度、小幅度、均匀提插捻转，使患者产生柔和、舒适、持久的针感；每穴操作2~3分钟。②生物反馈治疗：采用3种类型的生物反馈治疗，即单纯电刺激、肌电触发电刺激和放松训练。a. 盆底神经肌肉电刺激：利用10~50Hz、200μs的波宽、0~100mA的电流来进行恰当的神经肌肉电刺激，目的是尽快让患者增强对盆底肌肉的本体感觉，增强神经的兴奋性，结合患者的家庭训练，让患者尽快掌握盆底肌肉收缩及放松的感觉。b. 盆底神经肌肉肌电触发电刺激：增加阈值的设定，患者可通过主动收缩达到阈值线而获得一次电刺激，加强盆底肌肉收缩、放松感觉的记忆。通过不断地重复收缩训练、电刺激，患者最终学会如何自主正确收缩盆底肌肉。c. 放松训练：以静息值的80%为第一次的阈值，进行多媒体放松训练，通过动画、音乐、数字等音频、视频的反馈形式，让患者了解如何放松、如何收缩，并且可以设定放松或者收缩的具体达到的值，逐渐降低阈值至2~4μV。

疗程：每日1次，每次留针30分钟，每周治疗5次。4周为1个疗程，共治疗20次。

注意事项：①背俞穴针刺过程中，须注意掌握深度，位于肺脏投影区的背俞穴以斜刺为宜，深度不宜超过1寸。②中髎、下髎深刺过程中，针感强烈，须向患者做好解释工作。

『推荐』

> 推荐建议：推荐毫针刺法结合生物反馈治疗盆底失弛缓综合征。[GRADE 2C]

解释：本《指南》小组共纳入相关文献1篇[47]，经综合分析，形成证据体发现，毫针刺法结合生物反馈疗法治疗盆底失弛缓综合征，可明显减轻腹痛和排便窒塞感，改善大便性状。但纳入的文献偏倚风险较高，证据体质量等级经GRADE评价后，因其纳入文献设计质量低、证据间接及不精确性，最终证据体质量等级为低。

方案二：深刺中髎、下髎穴

现代医学认为，骶神经根从骶后孔处穿出，受电刺激后兴奋传入纤维，经脊髓和脑桥反射后再作用于盆腔器官，从而调整尿便反射。排便动作受大脑皮层及腰骶部脊髓内低级中枢的调节，深刺中髎、下髎穴，可刺激低级中枢向上传导，出现排便意识。中髎、下髎穴位于腰骶部，骶骨前方即是直肠，通过深刺中髎、下髎穴，即能起到近治作用。

取穴：中髎（双侧）、下髎（双侧）。

针刺方法：选取直径0.38mm、长度75mm的毫针，与皮肤垂直进针，缓慢将针刺入，调整针尖方向，直至有沉紧且涩滞感，此时需用较大的指力方能将针缓慢推入骶后孔内。当无骨性阻挡时，即为成功刺入骶后孔的标志。针刺时如果反复多次未能刺入骶后孔，在确定定位准确的前提下，可将针身上提但不提出皮肤表面，再将针尖方向向内调整，可在骶后孔附近探寻以求刺入之处。针刺深度 2.5~2.8 寸。

疗程：每周 5 次，4 周为 1 个疗程。

注意事项：中髎、下髎穴的体表定位及针刺中是否能顺利进入孔内通道均有相当的难度，针刺中应缓慢进针，随时调整针刺方向，如遇骨质阻挡而不能顺利进针时，不可强行进针，避免弯针、断针的情况发生。

『推荐』

> 推荐建议：推荐深刺中髎、下髎穴治疗盆底失弛缓综合征。[GRADE 2D]

解释：本《指南》小组共纳入相关文献 1 篇[48]，经综合分析，形成证据体发现，深刺中髎、下髎穴治疗盆底失弛缓综合征，可有效缓解腹痛及大便窒塞感，改善大便性状。但纳入的文献偏倚风险较高，证据体质量等级经 GRADE 评价后，因其纳入文献设计质量低及不精确性，最终证据体质量等级为极低。

5.4 糖尿病性便秘

现代医学认为，糖尿病性便秘与大肠自主神经病变、高血糖、消化道激素分泌异常、肠道平滑肌病变、精神心理因素及大肠敏感性降低有关，是多种因素共同作用的结果。其临床发病率较高，病程通常较长，治疗难度较大。针灸治疗必须在积极控制原发病的基础上进行。可考虑服用润肠通便的药物辅助治疗。

方案：毫针刺法结合中药疗法

取穴：天枢（双侧）、上巨虚（双侧）、大肠俞（双侧）、胃俞（双侧）、足三里（双侧）、关元。

操作方法：①毫针刺法：采用平补平泻法，进针深度以得气为度，获针感后，留针 20 分钟，起针。②中药疗法：予以五仁润肠方加减（药物组成略）。

疗程：每日 1 次，1 周为 1 个疗程，每个疗程之间休息 2 日。

注意事项：针灸治疗过程中，继续治疗原发病（糖尿病），积极控制血糖。

『推荐』

> 推荐建议：推荐以毫针刺法结合中药疗法治疗糖尿病性便秘。[GRADE 2D]

解释：本《指南》小组共纳入相关文献 1 篇[49]，经综合分析，形成证据体发现，毫针刺法结合中药疗法治疗糖尿病性便秘，可改善患者的生活质量，增加自主排便的次数。但纳入的文献偏倚风险较高，证据体质量等级经 GRADE 评价后，因其纳入文献设计质量低及不精确性，最终证据体质量等级为极低。

参考文献

［1］中华医学会消化病学分会胃肠动力学组，外科学分会结直肠肛门外科学组．中国慢性便秘的诊治指南［J］．中华消化杂志，2007，27（9）：619－622.

［2］于阶平，沈志祥，罗和生．实用消化病学［M］．北京：科学出版社，2007.

［3］王崇文，谢勇，邹多武，等．慢性便秘的诊断与治疗［J］．中华消化杂志，2004，24（1）：41－46.

［4］王宝西，王茂贵．功能性便秘流行病学调查及临床分析［J］．实用儿科临床杂志，2003，18（4）：253－254.

［5］郭晓峰，柯美云，潘国宗，等．北京地区成人慢性便秘整群、分层、随机流行病学调查及其相关因素分析［J］．中华消化杂志，2002，22（9）：637－638.

［6］魏艳静，卞红磊．便秘的国内流行病学研究进展［J］．疾病控制杂志，2004，8（5）：449－451.

［7］叶飞，王巧民．慢性便秘的流行病学研究进展［J］．中国临床保健杂志，2010，13（6）：665－557.

［8］熊理守，陈曼湖，陈惠新，等．广东省社区人群慢性便秘的流行病学研究［J］．中华消化杂志，2004，20（6）：488－491.

［9］中华消化学会胃肠动力学组．我国慢性便秘的诊治指南［J］．中国全科医学，2005，8（2）：119－121.

［10］罗马委员会．功能性胃肠病罗马Ⅲ诊断标准［J］．胃肠病学，2006，11（12）：761－765.

［11］中华中医药学会脾胃病分会．慢性便秘中医诊疗共识意见［J］．北京中医药，2011，30（1）：3－7.

［12］钱蒙，汪毓敏，任叔阳，等．慢性便秘的中西医治疗近况［J］．结直肠肛门外科，2008，14（1）：68－70.

［13］张雪芳，徐桂华，陈金珍，等．便秘的病因及治疗进展［J］．中华全科医学，2009，7（11）：1229－1230.

［14］周丽荣，林征，林琳，等．功能性便秘患者肛门直肠动力学与精神心理因素的相关性分析［J］．中华消化杂志，2009，29（2）：132－133.

［15］Brandt LJ, Prather CM, Quigley EM, et al. Systematic review on the management of chronic constipation in North America［J］. Am J Gastroenterol, 2005, 100（1）：55.

［16］Ramkumar D, Rao SS. Efficacy and safety of traditional medical therapies for chronic constipation：systematic review［J］. Am J Gastroenterol, 2005, 100（4）：936.

［17］徐彰，柯美云．慢性便秘的药物治疗评价［J］．中国新药杂志，2004，13（5）：389.

［18］任继平，刘宾．便秘的药物治疗［J］．中国医院用药评价与分析，2004，4（6）：372.

［19］丁海英，高春环，许凯．新型胃肠双动力药物——伊托必利［J］．中国医院药学杂志，2004，24：103－105.

［20］Hamilton MJM. Probiotics and prebiotics in the elderly［J］. Postgrad Med J, 2004, 80（946）：447－451.

［21］陈睿．神阙穴敷贴治疗便秘［J］．中国针灸，2002，22（8）：5411.

［22］伦新．生大黄粉神阙贴敷治疗中风便秘75例［J］．中国中西医结合杂志，2000，20

（2）：119.

［23］梁仲惠，杜平，彭丽琼，等．慢性功能性便秘结肠水疗临床疗效观察［J］．现代消化及介入治疗，2008，13（1）：58－59.

［24］吴晓青．慢性便秘的治疗进展［J］．中国疗养医学，2011，20（1）：59－60.

［25］张永刚，李国栋．慢传输性便秘治疗进展［J］．中国中西医结合外科杂志，2010，16（4）：507－510.

［26］杨洁，徐少勇，石振玉，等．胃肠起搏对慢传输型便秘疗效观察［J］．郧阳医学院学报，2007，26（3）：158－159.

［27］郭晓峰，柯美云，王智凤，等．电子药丸对慢传输型功能性便秘的随机双盲对照研究［J］．基础医学与临床，2003，23（增刊）：108.

［28］刘志顺．深刺天枢穴治疗结肠慢转运性便秘30例［J］．上海针灸杂志，2005，24（10）：26.

［29］李栓格，杜桂珍，张桂花．艾炷灸通便穴治疗便秘的临床观察［J］．河北中医，2009，31（1）：24.

［30］傅传刚．便秘的手术治疗指征和手术方式选择［J］．中华胃肠外科杂志，2007，10（2）：109－110.

［31］万兴．深刺天枢穴配合电针治疗功能性便秘远期疗效观察［D］．南京中医药大学硕士学位论文，2010.

［32］杨德莉，刘志顺．深刺天枢治疗功能性便秘疗效观察［J］．北京中医药，2010，29（5）：366－368.

［33］王成伟，李宁．电针双侧天枢穴对功能性便秘患者自觉症状的影响及疗效满意度评价：一项单中心、前瞻性随机对照临床试验［J］．针刺研究，2010，35（10）：375－378.

［34］吕慧．耳穴贴压法治疗便秘［J］．北京中医药，2009，28（5）：316－318.

［35］张怡芝，温庆贵，薛秀娟，等．耳穴埋针治疗功能性便秘50例［J］．河北中医药学报，2000，15（2）：41.

［36］刘杰．耳压治疗习惯性便秘88例［J］．河北中医，2007，29（1）：25.

［37］张梅．耳穴压丸法治疗便秘42例［J］．云南中医学院学报，2004，27（3）：54.

［38］马瑶，刘红．耳穴贴压加针刺治疗便秘60例［J］．长春中医药大学学报，2007，23（3）：57.

［39］张维．深刺天枢穴治疗结肠慢转运性便秘疗效及安全性评价［J］．中医杂志，2006，47（2）：105－109.

［40］卢岱魏．深刺天枢穴加电针治疗慢传输型便秘的疗效观察［D］．南京中医药大学硕士学位论文，2009.

［41］段锦绣，彭唯娜．天枢穴深刺治疗结肠慢传输型便秘的疗效评价［J］．南京中医药大学学报，2009，25（11）：424－427.

［42］彭唯娜，秦澎湃．个体化深刺天枢治疗结肠慢传输型便秘疗效及安全性评价［J］．江苏中医药，2010，42（7）：43－45.

［43］田宁．热敏灸治疗慢传输型便秘疗效观察［J］．湖北中医杂志，2009，31（11）：67－69.

［44］张智龙，吉学群．电针支沟穴治疗便秘之气秘多中心随机对照研究［J］．中国针灸．2007，27（7）：475－479.

［45］吴淑雯．靳三针治疗老年功能性便秘临床研究［D］．广州中医药大学博士学位论文，2009.

［46］梁谊深，罗莎．指针配合穴位埋线治疗便秘型肠易激综合征疗效观察［J］．上海针灸杂志，2010，29（3）：168－170.

[47] 季新涛. 生物反馈结合针灸治疗盆底失弛缓所致便秘的临床研究 [D]. 南京中医药大学硕士学位论文, 2009.

[48] 王丽娟, 王玲玲, 张晨静. 深刺中髎、下髎穴治疗盆底失弛缓型便秘 [J]. 针灸临床杂志, 2010, 1 (26)：27 -29.

[49] 刘瑞云. 针刺结合中药治疗糖尿病性便秘38 例 [J]. 光明中医, 2009, 24 (4)：702 -705.

附　　录

1　本《指南》专家组成员和编写组成员

专家组成员

姓名	职称	所在单位
田丛豁	主任医师	中国中医科学院广安门医院
李国栋	主任医师	中国中医科学院广安门医院
王麟鹏	主任医师	首都医科大学附属北京中医医院
刘绍能	主任医师	中国中医科学院广安门医院
赵吉平	主任医师	北京中医药大学东直门医院
王丽萍	主任医师	北京中医药大学附属护国寺中医医院
王　寅	主任医师	中国中医科学院广安门医院
黄石玺	主任医师	中国中医科学院广安门医院
胡静清	主任医师	中国中医科学院广安门医院
王映辉	主任医师	中国中医科学院广安门医院

编写组成员

姓名	性别	学位	职称	专业	工作单位	课题中的分工
张　维	男	博士	副主任医师	针灸	中国中医科学院广安门医院	组长，总体设计，组织实施，全程负责指南的编制及成稿
刘保延	男	硕士	主任医师	针灸	中国中医科学院	总负责人，管理、组织指南的编写以及分配任务
刘志顺	男	博士	主任医师	针灸	中国中医科学院广安门医院	方法学指导
彭唯娜	女	本科	副主任医师	针灸	中国中医科学院广安门医院	指南主要编写人员
张　涛	男	硕士	住院医师	针灸	首都医科大学附属北京中医医院	GRADE 文献质量评价，参与指南编写
郑铜铃	男	硕士	住院医师	针灸	北京中医药大学	文献质量评价，文献数据提取
王　韵	女	硕士	住院医师	针灸	北京中医药大学	现代文献检索，文献质量评价，指南编写人员
裴　蓓	女	硕士	住院医师	针灸	北京中医药大学	现代文献检索，文献数据提取，文献质量评价
李颂伊	女	硕士	—	针灸	北京中医药大学	外文文献检索，文献数据提取
金英利	女	硕士	—	针灸	北京中医药大学	外文文献检索，文献数据提取

2　临床问题

问题中必须包括以下四大要素：

P：Patient　　　　　　病人

I：Intervention　　　　干预

C：Comparison　　　　比较

A：Outcomes　　　　　评价

2.1 共性问题

针灸治疗慢性便秘的最佳操作方法。

不同病理分型便秘的最佳针灸治疗方法。

不同人群慢性便秘的最佳针灸治疗方法。

不同中医辨证分型慢性便秘的最佳针灸治疗方法。

针灸治疗慢性便秘的各种注意事项。

针灸治疗慢性便秘的不良反应及禁忌证。

慢性便秘患者对针灸干预措施的耐受度。

针灸治疗慢性便秘的卫生经济学评价是否优于其他疗法？

2.2 个性问题

2.2.1 一般便秘人群

2.2.1.1 未确定具体类型的慢性便秘

针灸治疗慢性功能性便秘的操作方法、注意事项、适应证及禁忌证。

2.2.1.2 结肠慢传输型便秘

针灸治疗结肠慢传输型便秘的操作方法、注意事项、适应证及禁忌证。

2.2.1.3 出口梗阻型便秘

针灸治疗出口梗阻型便秘的操作方法、注意事项、适应证及禁忌证。

2.2.1.4 混合型便秘

针灸治疗混合型便秘的操作方法、注意事项、适应证及禁忌证。

2.2.2 特定便秘人群

2.2.2.1 不同中医辨证分型的慢性便秘

针灸治疗不同中医辨证分型的慢性便秘的操作方法、注意事项、适应证及禁忌证。

2.2.2.2 不同年龄患者的慢性便秘

针灸治疗不同年龄患者的慢性便秘的操作方法、注意事项、适应证及禁忌证。

2.2.2.3 不同性别患者的慢性便秘

针灸治疗不同性别患者的慢性便秘的操作方法、注意事项、适应证及禁忌证。

3 疗效评价指标的分级

据 GRADE（Grading of Recommendations Assessment, Development, and Evaluation）证据质量评价系统，结局指标的重要程度分为 1～9 共 9 个等级，其中 1～3 为 Not Important（对决策影响不大的结果），4～6 为 Important（影响决策的重要而非关键结果），7～9 为 Critical（影响决策的关键结果）。每级又分为三个数值，数值越大，重要性越大。据统计，所有针灸治疗慢性便秘的文献共涉及结局评价指标 21 个，根据以上原则，结合慢性便秘的临床研究特点，拟定结局指标的重要程度分级为：

9：患者对治疗的满意度；

8：暂缺；

7：治疗有效（痊愈）率；

6：结肠运转时间（CTT）；

5：生活质量评分（PAC－QOL）；

4：心理症状自评量表（SCL－90）；

3：包括 CCS 评分、大便形状，治疗后首次自主排便距治疗结束时间，自主排便次数差，治疗前后排便时间差异，治疗前后及治疗中症状总积分差，治疗前后 72 小时结肠标志物排出率差值比较，治疗前后粪便性状正常率，抑郁自评量表 SDS，焦虑自评量表 SAS，治疗前后排便速度差，治疗前后大便性状差，治疗前后排便难度积分差，治疗前后便意积分差，治疗前后排便间隔时间差，排便不尽感差值，排便频率评分差值，共 16 项。

4 检索范围、检索策略及结果

4.1 检索范围

4.1.1 古代文献

采用手工检索方式逐本翻阅指南组提供的 55 本针灸古籍，由 2 名研究生于中国中医科学院图书馆、军事医学图书馆及中国医学科学院图书馆中进行，其中有 3 本未找到相应版本，能找到原文的图书共 52 本。

4.1.2 针灸医家经验

古代：手工检索 33 位古代针灸医家的与针灸相关的 48 部著作。

近代：手工检索 15 位近代针灸专家的 31 部著作。

4.1.3 过刊

在中国中医药期刊文献数据库检索系统（中国中医科学院信息所研制）中进行，检索文献的年份为 1949～1983 年。

4.1.4 现刊

在 MEDLINE（1966～2012 年）、中国生物医学文献光盘数据库（CBM，1994～2012 年）、中文生物医学期刊全文数据库（CMCC，1994～2012 年）、CNKI（1994～2012 年）以及日韩相关文献的数据库中检索。配合手工检索，在《中国针灸》（1981～2012 年）、《针灸临床杂志》（1985～2006 年）、《上海针灸杂志》（1982～2012 年）、《针刺研究》（1976～2012 年）杂志中，检索从创刊年至 2012 年发表的相关文章，同时收集未发表的文献（包括针灸学会会议论文、研究生及博士论文等相关汇编等）或正在进行的研究结论等。

4.2 检索策略

检索词分为以下几类：

4.2.1 古代文献

Locate Disease：#1 后不利；#2 大便难；#3 不更衣；#4 秘结；#5 脾约；#6 阴结；#7 阳结；#8 不大便；#9 大便不通；#10 风秘；#11 气秘；#12 热秘；#13 寒秘；#14 湿秘；#15 虚秘；#16 热燥；#17 风燥；#18 结燥；#19 大便秘；#20 大便秘涩；#21 1－20/or。

Locate Intervention：#22 针刺；#23 针灸；#24 针；#25 灸；#26 火针；#27 燔针；#28 放血；#29 罐；#30 22－29/or。

#31 #21 and #30

4.2.2 近现代文献（中文）

Locate Disease：#1 便秘；#2 大便难；#3 秘结；#4 1－3/or。

Locate Intervention：#5 针刺；#6 针灸；#7 电针；#8 火针；#9 温针；#10 梅花针；#11 头针；#12 耳针；#13 耳穴；#14 耳压；#15 芒针；#16 灸；#17 放血；#18 罐；#19 穴位注射；#20 埋线；#21 皮内针；#22 5－21/or。

#23 #4 and #22

4.2.3 近现代文献（英文）

Locate Disease：#1 Constipation.

Locate Intervention：#2 Acupuncture；#3 Moxibustion；#4 Electroacupuncture；#5 Fire Needling；#6 Warm Needling；#7 Pyonex；#8 Scalp Acupuncture；#9 Auricular Acupuncture；#10 Elongated Needle；#11 Pricking Blood；#12 Cupping；#13 Point Injecting；#14 Catgut Embedding；#15 Intradermal Needling；#16 2－15/or.

#17 #1 and #16

4.2.4 近现代文献（韩文）

Locate Disease：#1변비；#2잔변감；#3배변곤란；#4대변비결；#5 1-4/or。

LocateIntervention：#6침술；#7침구；#8전기침；#9화침；#10매화침；#11두피침；#12이침；#13장침；#14뜸；#15사혈；#16부항；#17약침；#18 6-17/or。

#19 #5 and #18

4.3 检索结果

依据既定的文献检索策略，对古代文献、中文过刊文献、现代文献（包括中文、英文、日文、韩文等）及专家经验进行了相关的检索工作，最终选定576篇针灸治疗便秘的相关文献，包括近代专家经验条文4条。

最终结果如下表所示：

文献检索结果汇总表 （篇）

			相关文献	已剔除文献	未找到文献	总计
古代文献检索			106	103	3	0
中文过刊检索			0	0	0	0
专家经验检索（近代专家）			4	0	0	4
现代文献检索	中文	已发表	725	149	0	576
		未发表	0	0	0	0
	英文		63	56	7	0
	日文		25	25	0	0
	韩文		20	20	0	0

5 文献质量评估结论

5.1 证据概要表（Evidence Profile, EP）

Author（s）：

Date：2011－06－06

Question：手针＋穴位注射 VS 药物 for 慢性便秘

Settings：

Bibliography：针灸 for 慢性便秘．Cochrane Database of Systematic Reviews［Year］，Issue［Issue］．

Quality assessment							No of patients		Effect		Quality	Importance
No of studies	Design	Limitations	Inconsistency	Indirectness	Imprecision	Other considerations	手针＋穴位注射 VS 药物	control	Relative (95% CI)	Absolute		
总有效率（follow–up mean 4 weeks; revman）												
1	randomised trials	serious[1]	no serious inconsistency[2]	serious[3]	no serious imprecision	reporting bias[2]	22/23 (95.7%)	15/22 (68.2%)	RR 1.4 (1.04 to 1.89)	273 more per 1000 (from 27 more to 607 more)	VERY LOW	CRITICAL
								68.2%		273 more per 1000 (from 27 more to 607 more)		

1 试验天生育法不足；报告未分析试验本身存在的偏移可能性。

2 只有一个试验研究。

3 主观测量指标。

Author（s）：

Date：2011－06－06

Question：指针＋穴位注射 VS 药物 for 慢性便秘

Settings：

Bibliography：针灸 for 慢性便秘. Cochrane Database of Systematic Reviews [Year], Issue [Issue] .

No of studies	Quality assessment						No of patients		Effect		Quality	Importance
	Design	Limitations	Inconsistency	Indirectness	Imprecision	Other considerations	指针＋穴位注射 VS 药物	control	Relative (95% CI)	Absolute		
总有效率 (follow－up mean 30 days; revman)												
1	randomised trials	serious[1]	no serious inconsistency	serious[2]	no serious imprecision	reporting bias[3]	32/35 (91.4%)	22/32 (68.8%)	RR 1.33 (1.03 to 1.72)	227 more per 1000 (from 21 more to 495 more)	VERY LOW	CRITICAL
								68.8%		227 more per 1000 (from 21 more to 495 more)		

1 随机分组人员参与纳入病人；利益相关；未实施盲法。

2 结局指标为主观性间接证据。

3 只有一篇文献。

Author（s）:

Date: 2011 – 06 – 06

Question: 指针 + 穴位埋线 VS 药物 for 慢性便秘

Settings:

Bibliography: 针灸 for 慢性便秘. Cochrane Database of Systematic Reviews [Year], Issue [Issue].

Quality assessment							Summary of findings					
							No of patients		Effect			
No of studies	Design	Limitations	Inconsistency	Indirectness	Imprecision	Other considerations	指针 + 穴位埋线 VS 药物	control	Relative (95% CI)	Absolute	Quality	Importance
总有效率 (follow – up mean 5 weeks; revman)												
1	randomised trials	serious[1]	no serious inconsistency	serious[2]	no serious imprecision	reporting bias[3]	14/38 (36.8%)	21/30 (70%)	RR 1.32 (1.02 to 1.69)	224 more per 1000 (from 14 more to 483 more)	VERY LOW	CRITICAL
								70%		224 more per 1000 (from 14 more to 483 more)		

1 盲法天生设计缺陷；未分析试验本身存在的偏移可能性。

2 主观指标。

3 只有一个试验。

Author（s）:

Date: 2011 – 06 – 06

Question: 温针 + 中药汤剂 VS 药物 for 慢性便秘

Settings:

Bibliography: 针灸 for 慢性便秘. Cochrane Database of Systematic Reviews [Year], Issue [Issue].

总有效率（follow – up mean 10 days; revman）

No of studies	Quality assessment						Summary of findings				Quality	Importance
	Design	Limitations	Inconsistency	Indirectness	Imprecision	Other considerations	No of patients		Effect			
							温针 + 中药汤剂 VS 药物	control	Relative (95% CI)	Absolute		
1	randomised trials	serious[1]	no serious inconsistency	serious[2]	no serious imprecision	reporting bias[3]	29/30 (96.7%)	22/30 (73.3%)	RR 1.32 (1.05 to 1.65)	235 more per 1000 (from 37 more to 477 more)	VERY LOW	CRITICAL
								73.3%		235 more per 1000 (from 37 more to 476 more)		

1 盲法缺陷；分配隐藏缺陷。

2 结局指标以主观为主。

3 只有一篇文献。

Author (s)：

Date：2011 – 06 – 06

Question：耳穴压豆 VS 药物 for 慢性便秘

Settings：

Bibliography：针灸 for 慢性便秘. Cochrane Database of Systematic Reviews [Year]，Issue [Issue].

	Quality assessment						No of patients		Effect		Quality	Importance
No of studies	Design	Limitations	Inconsistency	Indirectness	Imprecision	Other considerations	耳穴压豆 VS 药物	control	Relative (95% CI)	Absolute		
有效率（follow – up mean 8 weeks；revman）												
1	randomised trials	serious¹	no serious inconsistency	serious²	no serious imprecision	reporting bias³	27/30 (90%)	25/30 (83.3%)	RR 1.08 (0.88 to 1.32)	67 more per 1000 (from 100 fewer to 267 more)	VERY LOW	CRITICAL
								83.3%		67 more per 1000 (from 100 fewer to 267 more)		
首次排便时间（follow – up mean 8 weeks；Better indicated by lower values）												
1	randomised trials	serious¹	no serious inconsistency	no serious indirectness	no serious imprecision	reporting bias³	30	30	–	SMD 0.79 lower (1.31 to 0.26 lower)	LOW	NOT IMPORTANT
治疗前后总积分差（follow – up mean 8 weeks；Better indicated by lower values）												
1	randomised trials	serious¹	no serious inconsistency	serious²	no serious imprecision	reporting bias³	30	30	–	SMD 0.71 higher (0.19 to 1.24 higher)	VERY LOW	NOT IMPORTANT

Summary of findings

续表

No of studies	Quality assessment						No of patients		Summary of findings			
	Design	Limitations	Inconsistency	Indirectness	Imprecision	Other considerations	耳穴压豆 VS 药物	control	Effect		Quality	Importance
									Relative (95% CI)	Absolute		
治疗前后排便时间间差 (follow – up mean 8 weeks; Better indicated by lower values)												
1	randomised trials	serious[1]	no serious inconsistency	no serious indirectness	no serious imprecision	reporting bias[3]	30	30	–	SMD 0.3 higher (0.21 lower to 0.81 higher)	LOW	NOT IMPORTANT
治疗前后排便速度差值 (follow – up mean 8 weeks; Better indicated by lower values)												
1	randomised trials	serious[1]	no serious inconsistency	no serious indirectness	no serious imprecision	reporting bias[3]	30	30	–	SMD 1.06 higher (0.52 to 1.6 higher)	LOW	NOT IMPORTANT
治疗前后大便性状差 (follow – up mean 8 weeks; Better indicated by lower values)												
1	randomised trials	serious[1]	no serious inconsistency	serious[2]	no serious imprecision	reporting bias[3]	30	30	–	SMD 0.63 higher (0.11 1.15 higher)	VERY LOW	NOT IMPORTANT
治疗前后排便难度积分差 (follow – up mean 8 weeks; Better indicated by lower values)												
1	randomised trials	serious[1]	no serious inconsistency	serious[2]	no serious imprecision	reporting bias[3]	30	30	–	SMD 0.11 higher (0.39 lower to 0.62 higher)	VERY LOW	NOT IMPORTANT
治疗前后便意积分差 (follow – up mean 8 weeks; Better indicated by lower values)												
1	randomised trials	serious[1]	no serious inconsistency	serious[2]	no serious imprecision	reporting bias[3]	30	30	–	SMD 0.45 higher (0.06 lower to 0.97 higher)	VERY LOW	NOT IMPORTANT

1 分配隐藏；盲法缺陷。
2 结局以主观为主。
3 只有一个试验。

Author (s):

Date: 2011 – 06 – 06

Question: 手针 VS 手针 for 慢性便秘

Settings:

Bibliography: 针灸 for 慢性便秘. Cochrane Database of Systematic Reviews [Year], Issue [Issue].

有效率 (follow – up mean 3 weeks; revman)

No of studies	Quality assessment						No of patients		Effect		Quality	Importance
	Design	Limitations	Inconsistency	Indirectness	Imprecision	Other considerations	手针 VS 手针	control	Relative (95% CI)	Absolute		
1	randomised trials	serious[1]	no serious inconsistency	serious[2]	no serious imprecision[3]	reporting bias[4]	28/32 (87.5%)	24/30 (80%) 80%	RR 1.09 (0.88 to 1.37)	72 more per 1000 (from 96 fewer to 296 more) 72 more per 1000 (from 96 fewer to 296 more)	VERY LOW	CRITICAL

粪便性状正常率 (follow – up mean 3 weeks; revman)

| 1 | randomised trials | serious | no serious inconsistency | serious[2] | no serious imprecision[3] | reporting bias[4] | 15/32 (46.9%) | 12/30 (40%) 40% | RR 1.17 (0.66 to 2.08) | 68 more per 1000 (from 136 fewer to 432 more) 68 more per 1000 (from 136 fewer to 432 more) | VERY LOW | NOT IMPORTANT |

治疗前后症状总积分差 (follow – up mean 3 weeks; Better indicated by lower values)

| 1 | randomised trials | serious[1] | no serious inconsistency | serious[2] | no serious imprecision[3] | reporting bias[4] | 32 | 30 | – | SMD 0.43 higher (0.08 lower to 0.93 higher) | VERY LOW | NOT IMPORTANT |

治疗前后排便间隔时间差 (follow – up mean 3 weeks; Better indicated by lower values)

| 1 | randomised trials | serious[1] | no serious inconsistency | no serious indirectness | no serious imprecision[3] | reporting bias[4] | 32 | 30 | – | SMD 0 higher (0.5 lower to 0.5 higher) | LOW | NOT IMPORTANT |

续表

No of studies	Quality assessment						No of patients		Summary of findings			
	Design	Limitations	Inconsistency	Indirectness	Imprecision	Other considerations	手针 VS 手针	control	Effect		Quality	Importance
									Relative (95% CI)	Absolute		
治疗前后排便速度差（follow – up mean 3 weeks; Better indicated by lower values)												
1	randomised trials	serious[1]	no serious inconsistency	no serious indirectness	no serious imprecision[3]	reporting bias[4]	32	30	–	SMD 1. 53 higher (0. 96 to 2. 1 higher)	LOW	NOT IMPOR-TANT
治疗前后排便难度差（follow – up mean 3 weeks; Better indicated by lower values)												
1	randomised trials	serious[1]	no serious inconsistency	serious[2]	no serious imprecision[3]	reporting bias[4]	32	30	–	SMD 0. 31 lower (0. 81 lower to 0. 19 higher)	VERY LOW	NOT IMPOR-TANT
治疗前后排便性状差值（follow – up mean 3 weeks; Better indicated by lower values)												
1	randomised trials	serious[1]	no serious inconsistency	serious[2]	no serious imprecision[3]	reporting bias[4]	32	30	–	SMD 0. 62 higher (0. 11 to 1. 13 higher)	VERY LOW	NOT IMPOR-TANT
治疗前后便意差值（follow – up mean 3 weeks; Better indicated by lower values)												
1	randomised trials	serious[1]	no serious inconsistency	serious[2]	no serious imprecision[3]	reporting bias[4]	32	30	–	SMD 0 higher (0. 5 lower to 0. 5 higher)	VERY LOW	NOT IMPOR-TANT
治疗前后焦虑自评量 SAS 表差值（follow – up mean 3 weeks; Better indicated by lower values)												
1	randomised trials	serious[1]	no serious inconsistency	serious[2]	no serious imprecision[3]	reporting bias[4]	32	30	–	SMD 1. 61 higher (1. 03 to 2. 18 higher)	VERY LOW	NOT IMPOR-TANT

1 分配隐藏；盲法缺陷。
2 主观指标。
3 样本量小；可信区间宽。
4 只有一个试验纳入。

Author (s):

Date: 2011 – 06 – 06

Question: 灸法 VS 药物 for 慢性便秘

Settings:

Bibliography: 针灸 for 慢性便秘. Cochrane Database of Systematic Reviews [Year], Issue [Issue].

Quality assessment							No of patients		Summary of findings			
									Effect			
No of studies	Design	Limitations	Inconsistency	Indirectness	Imprecision	Other considerations	灸法 VS 药物	control	Relative (95% CI)	Absolute	Quality	Importance
总有效率 (follow-up mean 2 months; revman)												
1	randomised trials	serious[1]	no serious inconsistency	serious[2]	no serious imprecision[3]	reporting bias[4]	26/30 (86.7%)	16/30 (53.3%)	RR 1.62 (1.13 to 2.34)	331 more per 1000 (from 69 more to 715 more)	VERY LOW	CRITICAL
								53.3%		330 more per 1000 (from 69 more to 714 more)		

1 盲法、分配隐藏缺陷。
2 主观指标。
3 样本量小；可信区间宽。
4 只有一个试验被纳入。

Author (s)：

Date：2011 – 06 – 06

Question：电针 + 灸法 VS 电针 for 慢性便秘

Settings：

Bibliography：针灸 for 慢性便秘. Cochrane Database of Systematic Reviews [Year], Issue [Issue].

| | Quality assessment | | | | | | No of patients | | Summary of findings | | | |
| | | | | | | | | | Effect | | | |
No of studies	Design	Limitations	Inconsistency	Indirectness	Imprecision	Other considerations	电针 + 灸法 VS 电针	control	Relative (95% CI)	Absolute	Quality	Importance
有效率（follow – up mean 20 days；revman）												
1	randomised trials	no serious limitations	no serious inconsistency	serious	no serious imprecision[1]	reporting bias[2]	35/50 (70%)	26/50 (52%)	RR 1.35 (0.98 to 1.86)	182 more per 1000（from 10 fewer to 447 more）	LOW	CRITICAL
								52%		182 more per 1000（from 10 fewer to 447 more）		
治疗前后生活质量 PAC – QOL 差值（follow – up mean 20 days；Better indicated by lower values）												
1	randomised trials	no serious limitations	no serious inconsistency	serious[3]	no serious imprecision[1]	reporting bias[2]	50	50	–	SMD 0.53 higher (0.13 to 0.93 higher)	LOW	IMPORTANT
治疗前后心理症状评分 SCL – 90 差值（follow – up mean 20 days；Better indicated by lower values）												
1	randomised trials	no serious limitations	no serious inconsistency	serious[3]	no serious imprecision[1]	reporting bias[2]	50	50	–	SMD 0.19 higher (0.21 lower to 0.58 higher)	LOW	IMPORTANT

1 样本量小；95% CI 宽。

2 只有一个试验。

3 主观性指标。

Author (s):

Date: 2011 – 06 – 06

Question: 电针 VS sham needle for 慢性便秘

Settings:

Bibliography: 针灸 for 慢性便秘. Cochrane Database of Systematic Reviews [Year], Issue [Issue].

No of studies	Quality assessment						No of patients		Summary of findings		Quality	Importance
	Design	Limitations	Inconsistency	Indirectness	Imprecision	Other considerations	电针 VS sham needle	control	Effect			
									Relative (95% CI)	Absolute		

有效率 (follow – up mean 4 weeks; revman)

| 1 | randomised trials | no serious limitations | no serious inconsistency | serious[1] | no serious imprecision | reporting bias[2] | 119/126 (94.4%) | 79/129 (61.2%) | RR 1.54 (1.34 to 1.78) | 331 more per 1000 (from 208 more to 478 more) | LOW | CRITICAL |
| | | | | | | | | 61.2% | | 330 more per 1000 (from 208 more to 477 more) | | |

治疗 1 周症状积分差值 (follow – up mean 4 weeks; Better indicated by lower values)

| 1 | randomised trials | no serious limitations | no serious inconsistency | serious[1] | no serious imprecision | reporting bias[2] | 126 | 129 | – | SMD 8.25 higher (7.48 to 9.01 higher) | LOW | NOT IMPORTANT |

治疗 2 周症状积分差值 (follow – up mean 4 weeks; Better indicated by lower values)

| 1 | randomised trials | no serious limitations | no serious inconsistency | serious[1] | no serious imprecision | reporting bias[2] | 126 | 129 | – | SMD 11.47 higher (10.44 to 12.5 higher) | LOW | NOT IMPORTANT |

治疗 3 周症状积分差值 (follow – up mean 4 weeks; Better indicated by lower values)

| 1 | randomised trials | no serious limitations | no serious inconsistency | serious[1] | no serious imprecision | reporting bias[2] | 126 | 129 | – | SMD 17.27 higher (15.74 to 18.8 higher) | LOW | NOT IMPORTANT |

续表

No of studies	Quality assessment						No of patients		Summary of findings		Quality	Importance
	Design	Limitations	Inconsistency	Indirectness	Imprecision	Other considerations	电针 VS sham needle	control	Effect			
									Relative (95% CI)	Absolute		
治疗4周症状积分差值（follow – up mean 4 weeks；Better indicated by lower values）												
1	randomised trials	no serious limitations	no serious inconsistency	serious[1]	no serious imprecision	reporting bias[2]	126	129	–	SMD 24.81 higher (22.63 to 27 higher)	LOW	NOT IMPORTANT
治疗后1月随访症状积分差值（follow – up mean 4 weeks；Better indicated by lower values）												
1	randomised trials	no serious limitations	no serious inconsistency	serious[1]	no serious imprecision	reporting bias[2]	126	129	–	SMD 12.4 higher (11.29 to 13.52 higher)	LOW	NOT IMPORTANT
治疗后3月随访症状积分差值（follow – up mean 4 weeks；Better indicated by lower values）												
1	randomised trials	no serious limitations	no serious inconsistency	serious[1]	no serious imprecision	reporting bias[2]	126	129	–	SMD 11.73 higher (10.68 to 12.79 higher)	LOW	NOT IMPORTANT
治疗前后72小时结肠标志物排除率差值（follow – up mean 4 weeks；Better indicated by lower values）												
1	randomised trials	no serious limitations	no serious inconsistency	no serious indirectness	no serious imprecision	reporting bias[2]	126	129	–	SMD 1.73 higher (1.44 to 2.02 higher)	MODERATE	NOT IMPORTANT

1 主观性指标。
2 只有一个试验纳入。

Author (s):

Date: 2011 – 06 – 06

Question: 针刺+灸法 VS 生物反馈 for 慢性便秘

Settings:

Bibliography: 针灸 for 慢性便秘. Cochrane Database of Systematic Reviews [Year], Issue [Issue].

No of studies	Quality assessment						No of patients		Summary of findings		Quality	Importance
	Design	Limitations	Inconsistency	Indirectness	Imprecision	Other considerations	针刺+灸法 VS 生物反馈	control	Effect			
									Relative (95% CI)	Absolute		
有效率 (follow – up mean 2 weeks; revman)												
1	randomised trials	serious[1]	no serious inconsistency	serious[1]	no serious imprecision[2]	reporting bias[3]	10/20 (50%)	6/20 (30%)	RR 1.67 (0.75 to 3.71)	201 more per 1000 (from 75 fewer to 813 more)	VERY LOW	CRITICAL
								30%		201 more per 1000 (from 75 fewer to 813 more)		
治疗前后 PAC – QOL 评分差值 (follow – up mean 2 weeks; Better indicated by lower values)												
1	randomised trials	serious[4]	no serious inconsistency	serious[1]	serious[2]	reporting bias[3]	20	20	–	SMD 0.16 higher (0.46 lower to 0.78 higher)	VERY LOW	IMPORTANT

1 主观指标。

2 样本量小。

3 只有一篇文献纳入。

4 分配隐藏；盲法缺陷。

Author (s):

Date: 2011 – 06 – 06

Question: 针刺 + 灸法 + 生物反馈 VS 生物反馈 for 慢性便秘

Settings:

Bibliography: 针灸 for 慢性便秘. Cochrane Database of Systematic Reviews [Year], Issue [Issue].

有效率 (follow – up mean 2 weeks; revman)

| No of studies | Quality assessment | | | | | | No of patients | | Effect | | Quality | Importance |
	Design	Limitations	Inconsistency	Indirectness	Imprecision	Other considerations	针刺+灸法+生物反馈 VS 生物反馈	control	Relative (95% CI)	Absolute		
1	randomised trials	serious[1]	no serious inconsistency	serious[2]	no serious imprecision[3]	reporting bias[4]	13/20 (65%)	6/20 (30%)	RR 2.17 (1.03 to 4.55)	351 more per 1000 (from 9 more to 1065 more)	VERY LOW	CRITICAL
								30%		351 more per 1000 (from 9 more to 1065 more)		

治疗前后 PAC – QOL 评分差值 (follow – up mean 2 weeks; Better indicated by lower values)

No of studies	Design	Limitations	Inconsistency	Indirectness	Imprecision	Other considerations	针刺+灸法+生物反馈 VS 生物反馈	control	Relative (95% CI)	Absolute	Quality	Importance
1	randomised trials	serious[1]	no serious inconsistency	serious[2]	no serious imprecision[3]	reporting bias[4]	20	20	-	SMD 0.4 higher (0.22 lower to 1.03 higher)	VERY LOW	IMPORTANT

1 分配隐藏；盲法缺陷。

2 主观指标。

3 样本量小。

4 只有一篇文献纳入。

Author（s）：

Date：2011 – 06 – 06

Question：针刺 + 灸法 + 生物反馈 VS 针刺 + 灸法 for 慢性便秘

Settings：

Bibliography：针灸 for 慢性便秘．Cochrane Database of Systematic Reviews［Year］，Issue［Issue］．

No of studies	Quality assessment						Summary of findings					
	Design	Limitations	Inconsistency	Indirectness	Imprecision	Other considerations	No of patients		Effect		Quality	Importance
							针刺 + 灸法 + 生物反馈 VS 针刺 + 灸法	control	Relative (95% CI)	Absolute		
有效率（follow – up mean 2 weeks；revman）												
1	randomised trials	serious[1]	no serious inconsistency	serious[2]	no serious imprecision[3]	reporting bias[4]	13/20 (65%)	10/20 (50%)	RR 1.3 (0.75 to 2.24)	150 more per 1000 (from 125 fewer to 620 more)	VERY LOW	CRITICAL
								50%		150 more per 1000 (from 125 fewer to 620 more)		
治疗前后 PAC – QOL 评分差值（follow – up mean 2 weeks；Better indicated by lower values）												
1	randomised trials	serious[1]	no serious inconsistency	serious[2]	no serious imprecision[3]	reporting bias[4]	20	20	–	SMD 0.28 higher (0.34 lower to 0.9 higher)	VERY LOW	IMPORTANT

1 盲法、分配隐藏缺陷。
2 主观指标。
3 样本量小。
4 只纳入一篇文献。

Author (s):

Date: 2011 – 06 – 06

Question: 穴位埋线 VS 药物 for 慢性便秘

Settings:

Bibliography: 针灸 for 慢性便秘. Cochrane Database of Systematic Reviews [Year], Issue [Issue].

No of studies	Design	Limitations	Inconsistency	Indirectness	Imprecision	Other considerations	穴位埋线 VS 药物	control	Relative (95% CI)	Absolute	Quality	Importance
			Quality assessment				No of patients		Effect			
治疗2周后有效率（follow – up mean 2 weeks; revman）												
2	randomised trials	serious[1]	no serious inconsistency	serious[2]	no serious imprecision	none	55/60 (91.7%)	44/60 (73.3%) 73.3%	RR 1.24 (1.05 to 1.47)	176 more per 1000 (from 37 more to 345 more) 176 more per 1000 (from 37 more to 345 more)	LOW	CRITICAL
治疗2周后有效率 – 脾俞 + 大肠俞埋线 VS 莫沙必利（follow – up mean 2 weeks; revman）												
1	randomised trials	serious[3]	no serious inconsistency	serious[2]	serious[1]	reporting bias[4]	27/30 (90%)	23/30 (76.7%) 76.7%	RR 1.17 (0.93 to 1.48)	130 more per 1000 (from 54 fewer to 368 more) 130 more per 1000 (from 54 fewer to 368 more)	VERY LOW	CRITICAL
治疗2周后有效率 – 天枢 + 大肠俞 + 关元 + 足三里 VS 莫沙必利（follow – up mean 2 weeks; revman）												
1	randomised trials	serious[1]	no serious inconsistency	serious[2]	no serious imprecision	reporting bias[4]	28/30 (93.3%)	21/30 (70%) 70%	RR 1.33 (1.04 to 1.72)	231 more per 1000 (from 28 more to 504 more) 231 more per 1000 (from 28 more to 504 more)	VERY LOW	CRITICAL
治疗4周后有效率（follow – up mean 4 weeks; revman）												
1	randomised trials	serious[3]	no serious inconsistency	serious[2]	no serious imprecision	reporting bias[4]	26/30 (86.7%)	16/30 (53.3%) 53.3%	RR 1.62 (1.13 to 2.34)	331 more per 1000 (from 69 more to 715 more) 330 more per 1000 (from 69 more to 714 more)	VERY LOW	CRITICAL

Summary of findings

续表

No of studies	Design			Quality assessment				No of patients		Summary of findings		Quality	Importance
		Limitations	Inconsistency	Indirectness	Imprecision	Other considerations		穴位埋线 VS 药物	control	Effect			
										Relative (95% CI)	Absolute		
治疗结束后 30 天有效率 (follow – up mean 30 days; revman)													
1	randomised trials	serious[1]	no serious inconsistency	serious[2]	no serious imprecision	reporting bias[4]		82/87 (94.3%)	1/94 (1.1%)	RR 88.6 (12.6 to 622.85)	932 more per 1000 (from 123 more to 6615 more)	VERY LOW	CRITICAL
									1.1%		964 more per 1000 (from 128 more to 6840 more)		
治疗 1 次结束后 3 个月有效率 (follow – up mean 3 months; revman)													
1	randomised trials	serious[1]	no serious inconsistency	serious[2]	no serious imprecision	reporting bias[4]		82/87 (94.3%)	1/94 (1.1%)	RR 88.6 (12.6 to 622.85)	932 more per 1000 (from 123 more to 6615 more)	VERY LOW	CRITICAL
									1.1%		964 more per 1000 (from 128 more to 6840 more)		
排便间隔时间改善率 (follow – up mean 4 weeks; revman)													
1	randomised trials	serious[3]	no serious inconsistency	no serious indirectness	no serious imprecision	reporting bias[4]		25/28 (89.3%)	26/29 (89.7%)	RR 1 (0.83 to 1.19)	0 fewer per 1000 (from 152 fewer to 170 more)	LOW	NOT IMPORTANT
									89.7%		0 fewer per 1000 (from 152 fewer to 170 more)		
排便时间改善率 (follow – up mean 4 weeks; revman)													
1	randomised trials	serious[3]	no serious inconsistency	no serious indirectness	no serious imprecision	reporting bias[4]		18/21 (85.7%)	14/24 (58.3%)	RR 1.47 (1 to 2.15)	274 more per 1000 (from 0 more to 671 more)	LOW	NOT IMPORTANT
									58.3%		274 more per 1000 (from 0 more to 670 more)		
粪便性质改善率 (follow – up mean 4 weeks; revman)													
1	randomised trials	serious[3]	no serious inconsistency	serious[2]	no serious imprecision	reporting bias[4]		22/28 (78.6%)	17/27 (63%)	RR 1.25 (0.88 to 1.77)	157 more per 1000 (from 76 fewer to 485 more)	VERY LOW	NOT IMPORTANT
									63%		157 more per 1000 (from 76 fewer to 485 more)		

续表

No of studies	Quality assessment						No of patients		Summary of findings		Quality	Importance
	Design	Limitations	Inconsistency	Indirectness	Imprecision	Other considerations	穴位埋线 VS 药物	control	Effect			
									Relative (95% CI)	Absolute		
排便困难程度改善率 (follow - up mean 4 weeks; revman)												
1	randomised trials	serious[3]	no serious inconsistency	serious[2]	no serious imprecision	reporting bias[4]	18/30 (60%)	9/30 (30%)	RR 2 (1.08 to 3.72)	300 more per 1000 (from 24 more to 816 more)	VERY LOW	NOT IMPORTANT
								30%		300 more per 1000 (from 24 more to 816 more)		
兼症改善率 (follow - up mean 4 weeks; revman)												
1	randomised trials	serious[3]	no serious inconsistency	serious[2]	no serious imprecision	reporting bias[4]	20/26 (76.9%)	16/29 (55.2%)	RR 1.39 (0.94 to 2.06)	215 more per 1000 (from 33 fewer to 585 more)	VERY LOW	NOT IMPORTANT
								55.2%		215 more per 1000 (from 33 fewer to 585 more)		
治疗前后大便性状差值 (follow - up mean 2 weeks; Better indicated by lower values)												
1	randomised trials	serious[1]	no serious inconsistency	serious[2]	no serious imprecision	reporting bias[4]	30	30	–	SMD 1.31 higher (0.75 to 1.87 higher)	VERY LOW	NOT IMPORTANT
治疗前后每周排便次数差值 (follow - up mean 2 weeks; Better indicated by lower values)												
1	randomised trials	serious[1]	no serious inconsistency	no serious indirectness	no serious imprecision	reporting bias[4]	30	30	–	SMD 0.21 lower (0.71 lower to 0.3 higher)	LOW	NOT IMPORTANT
治疗 4 次结束后 3 个月有效率 (follow - up mean 3 months; revman)												
1	randomised trials	no serious limitations	no serious inconsistency	serious[2]	no serious imprecision	reporting bias[4]	120/132 (90.9%)	107/132 (81.1%)	RR 1.12 (1.02 to 1.24)	97 more per 1000 (from 16 more to 195 more)	LOW	CRITICAL

续表

治疗结束后6个月有效率（follow-up mean 6 months; revman）

No of studies	Quality assessment						No of patients		Effect		Quality	Importance
	Design	Limitations	Inconsistency	Indirectness	Imprecision	Other considerations	穴位埋线 VS 药物	control	Relative (95% CI)	Absolute		
1	randomised trials	no serious limitations	no serious inconsistency	serious[2]	no serious imprecision	reporting bias[4]	118/132 (89.4%)	94/132 (71.2%)	RR 1.26 (1.11 to 1.42)	185 more per 1000 (from 78 more to 299 more)	LOW	CRITICAL

1 分配隐藏及盲法缺陷。
2 主观性指标。
3 分配隐藏缺陷。
4 只纳入一篇文献。

Author（s）：

Date：2011 – 06 – 06

Question: 手针 VS 药物 for 慢性便秘

Settings:

Bibliography: 针灸 for 慢性便秘. Cochrane Database of Systematic Reviews [Year]，Issue [Issue].

开始治疗1个月后总有效率（revman）

No of studies	Quality assessment						No of patients		Effect		Quality	Importance
	Design	Limitations	Inconsistency	Indirectness	Imprecision	Other considerations	手针 VS 药物	control	Relative (95% CI)	Absolute		
2	randomised trials	serious[1]	serious[2]	serious[3]	no serious imprecision	none	100/105 (95.2%)	91/102 (89.2%) 88.7%	RR 1.07 (0.96 to 1.19)	62 more per 1000 (from 36 fewer to 170 more) 62 more per 1000 (from 35 fewer to 169 more)	VERY LOW	CRITICAL

续表

No of studies	Quality assessment						No of patients		Summary of findings		Quality	Importance
									Effect			
	Design	Limitations	Inconsistency	Indirectness	Imprecision	Other considerations	手针 VS 药物	control	Relative (95% CI)	Absolute		
开始治疗1个月后总有效率 - 手针背俞穴 VS 麻子仁丸 (follow – up mean 3 weeks; revman)												
1	randomised trials	no serious limitations	no serious inconsistency	serious[3]	no serious imprecision	reporting bias[4]	44/45 (97.8%)	36/42 (85.7%) / 85.7%	RR 1.14 (1 to 1.3)	120 more per 1000 (from 0 more to 257 more) / 120 more per 1000 (from 0 more to 257 more)	LOW	CRITICAL
开始治疗1个月后有效率 - 手针三其穴 VS 西沙必利 + 麻仁润肠丸 (follow – up mean 15 days; revman)												
1	randomised trials	serious[1]	no serious inconsistency	serious[3]	no serious imprecision	reporting bias[4]	56/60 (93.3%)	55/60 (91.7%) / 91.7%	RR 1.02 (0.92 to 1.13)	18 more per 1000 (from 73 fewer to 119 more) / 18 more per 1000 (from 73 fewer to 119 more)	VERY LOW	CRITICAL
开始治疗1个月后痊愈率 (follow – up mean 3 weeks; revman)												
1	randomised trials	no serious limitations	no serious inconsistency	serious[3]	no serious imprecision	reporting bias[5]	29/45 (64.4%)	15/42 (35.7%) / 35.7%	RR 1.8 (1.14 to 2.86)	286 more per 1000 (from 50 more to 664 more) / 286 more per 1000 (from 50 more to 664 more)	LOW	CRITICAL
开始治疗4个月后总有效率 (follow – up mean 3 weeks; revman)												
1	randomised trials	no serious limitations	no serious inconsistency	serious[3]	no serious imprecision	reporting bias[5]	45/45 (100%)	25/42 (59.5%) / 59.5%	RR 1.67 (1.3 to 2.14)	399 more per 1000 (from 179 more to 679 more) / 399 more per 1000 (from 178 more to 678 more)	LOW	CRITICAL
开始治疗4个月后痊愈率 (follow – up mean 3 weeks; revman)												
1	randomised trials	no serious limitations	no serious inconsistency	serious[3]	no serious imprecision	reporting bias[5]	35/45 (77.8%)	11/42 (26.2%) / 26.2%	RR 2.97 (1.75 to 5.05)	516 more per 1000 (from 196 more to 1061 more) / 516 more per 1000 (from 197 more to 1061 more)	LOW	CRITICAL

No of studies	Quality assessment						No of patients		Summary of findings		Quality	Importance
	Design	Limitations	Inconsistency	Indirectness	Imprecision	Other considerations	手针 VS 药物	control	Effect			
									Relative (95% CI)	Absolute		
治疗10次便秘评分差值（follow – up mean 20 days；Better indicated by lower values）												
1	randomised trials	no serious limitations	no serious inconsistency	serious[3]	no serious imprecision	reporting bias[5]	35	35	–	SMD 0.94 higher (0.45 to 1.44 higher)	LOW	NOT IMPORTANT
治疗20次便秘评分差值（follow – up mean 20 days；Better indicated by lower values）												
1	randomised trials	no serious limitations	no serious inconsistency	serious[3]	no serious imprecision	reporting bias[5]	35	35	–	SMD 3.68 higher (2.42 to 4.94 higher)	LOW	NOT IMPORTANT

1 盲法、分配隐藏缺陷。
2 去掉低质量、权重大文献后结果逆转。
3 主观指标。
4 只有一篇文献纳入亚组。
5 只有一篇文章纳入。

Author (s):

Date: 2011－06－06

Question: 电针 VS 电针 for 慢性便秘

Settings:

Bibliography: 针灸 for 慢性便秘. Cochrane Database of Systematic Reviews [Year], Issue [Issue].

No of studies	Design	Quality assessment					No of patients		Summary of findings		Quality	Importance
		Limitations	Inconsistency	Indirectness	Imprecision	Other considerations	电针 VS 电针	control	Effect			
									Relative (95% CI)	Absolute		
治疗 1 周后排便次数差值 (follow－up mean 4 weeks; Better indicated by lower values)												
1	randomised trials	no serious limitations	no serious inconsistency	no serious indirectness	no serious imprecision	reporting bias[1]	48	24	－	SMD 0.81 higher (0.3 to 1.32 higher)	MODERATE	NOT IMPORTANT
治疗 2 周后排便次数差值 (follow－up mean 4 weeks; Better indicated by lower values)												
1	randomised trials	no serious limitations	no serious inconsistency	no serious indirectness	no serious imprecision	reporting bias[1]	48	24	－	SMD 0.92 higher (0.41 to 1.43 higher)	MODERATE	NOT IMPORTANT
治疗 3 周后排便次数差值 (follow－up mean 4 weeks; Better indicated by lower values)												
1	randomised trials	no serious limitations	no serious inconsistency	no serious indirectness	no serious imprecision	reporting bias[1]	48	24	－	SMD 1.09 higher (0.57 to 1.62 higher)	MODERATE	NOT IMPORTANT
治疗 4 周后排便次数差值 (follow－up mean 4 weeks; Better indicated by lower values)												
2	randomised trials	no serious limitations	serious[2]	no serious indirectness	no serious imprecision	none	86	45	－	SMD 0.93 higher (0.13 lower to 1.98 higher)	MODERATE	NOT IMPORTANT
治疗结束后 4 周排便次数差值 (follow－up mean 4 weeks; Better indicated by lower values)												
1	randomised trials	no serious limitations	no serious inconsistency	no serious indirectness	no serious imprecision	reporting bias[1]	48	24	－	SMD 1.44 higher (0.89 to 1.98 higher)	MODERATE	NOT IMPORTANT
治疗结束后 12 周排便次数差值 (follow－up mean 4 weeks; Better indicated by lower values)												
1	randomised trials	no serious limitations	no serious inconsistency	no serious indirectness	no serious imprecision	reporting bias[1]	48	24	－	SMD 0.94 higher (0.42 to 1.45 higher)	MODERATE	NOT IMPORTANT

No of studies	Quality assessment						No of patients		Summary of findings		Quality	Importance
	Design	Limitations	Inconsistency	Indirectness	Imprecision	Other considerations	电针 VS 电针	control	Effect Relative (95% CI)	Absolute		
治疗结束后 6 个月排便次数差值（follow – up mean 4 weeks；Better indicated by lower values）												
1	randomised trials	no serious limitations	no serious inconsistency	no serious indirectness	no serious imprecision	reporting bias[1]	48	24	–	SMD 1.31 higher (0.77 to 1.85 higher)	MODERATE	NOT IMPORTANT
治疗 1 周便秘评分差值（follow – up mean 4 weeks；Better indicated by lower values）												
2	randomised trials	no serious limitations	no serious inconsistency	serious[3]	no serious imprecision	none	78	54	–	SMD 0.23 higher (0.14 lower to 0.6 higher)	MODERATE	NOT IMPORTANT
治疗 1 周便秘评分差值 – 深刺天枢 VS 浅刺天枢（follow – up mean 4 weeks；Better indicated by lower values）												
1	randomised trials	no serious limitations	no serious inconsistency	serious[3]	no serious imprecision	reporting bias[1]	48	24	–	SMD 0.42 higher (0.08 to 0.91 higher)	LOW	NOT IMPORTANT
治疗 1 周便秘评分差值 – 低频电针 VS 高频电针（follow – up mean 4 weeks；Better indicated by lower values）												
1	randomised trials	no serious limitations	no serious inconsistency	serious[3]	no serious imprecision	reporting bias[1]	30	30	–	SMD 0.04 higher (0.47 lower to 0.54 higher)	LOW	NOT IMPORTANT
治疗 2 周便秘评分差值（follow – up mean 4 weeks；Better indicated by lower values）												
2	randomised trials	no serious limitations	no serious inconsistency	serious[3]	no serious imprecision	none	78	54	–	SMD 0.18 higher (0.17 lower to 0.53 higher)	MODERATE	NOT IMPORTANT
治疗 2 周便秘评分差值 – 深刺天枢 VS 浅刺天枢（follow – up mean 4 weeks；Better indicated by lower values）												
1	randomised trials	no serious limitations	no serious inconsistency	serious[3]	no serious imprecision	reporting bias[1]	48	24	–	SMD 0.35 higher (0.15 lower to 0.84 higher)	LOW	NOT IMPORTANT

43

续表

No of studies	Quality assessment						No of patients		Summary of findings			Importance
	Design	Limitations	Inconsistency	Indirectness	Imprecision	Other considerations	电针 VS 电针	control	Effect		Quality	
									Relative (95% CI)	Absolute		
治疗 2 周便秘评分差值 电针 VS 低频电针（follow－up mean 4 weeks；Better indicated by lower values）												
1	randomised trials	no serious limitations	no serious inconsistency	serious[3]	no serious imprecision	reporting bias[1]	30	30	–	SMD 0 higher（0.51 lower to 0.51 higher）	LOW	NOT IMPORTANT
治疗 3 周便秘评分差值（follow－up mean 4 weeks；Better indicated by lower values）												
2	randomised trials	no serious limitations	no serious inconsistency	serious[3]	no serious imprecision	none	78	54	–	SMD 1.1 higher（0.79 lower to 2.99 higher）	MODERATE	NOT IMPORTANT
治疗 3 周便秘评分差值 深刺天枢 VS 浅刺天枢（follow－up mean 4 weeks；Better indicated by lower values）												
1	randomised trials	no serious limitations	no serious inconsistency	serious[3]	no serious imprecision	reporting bias[1]	48	24	–	SMD 2.07 higher（1.47 to 2.67 higher）	LOW	NOT IMPORTANT
治疗 3 周便秘评分差值 低频电针 VS 高频电针（follow－up mean 4 weeks；Better indicated by lower values）												
1	randomised trials	no serious limitations	no serious inconsistency	serious[3]	no serious imprecision	reporting bias[1]	30	30	–	SMD 0.14 higher（0.37 lower to 0.65 higher）	LOW	NOT IMPORTANT
治疗 4 周便秘评分差值（follow－up mean 4 weeks；Better indicated by lower values）												
5	randomised trials	no serious limitations	no serious inconsistency	serious[3]	no serious imprecision	none	146	115	–	SMD 0.57 higher（0.21 to 0.92 higher）	MODERATE	NOT IMPORTANT
治疗 4 周便秘评分差值 深刺天枢 VS 浅刺天枢（follow－up mean 4 weeks；Better indicated by lower values）												
4	randomised trials	no serious limitations	no serious inconsistency	serious[3]	no serious imprecision	reporting bias[1]	116	85	–	SMD 0.72 higher（0.42 to 1.02 higher）	LOW	NOT IMPORTANT

治疗4周便秘评分差值 － 低频电针 VS 高频电针（follow－up mean 4 weeks；Better indicated by lower values）

治疗结束后4周便秘评分差值（follow－up mean 4 weeks；Better indicated by lower values）

治疗结束后12周便秘评分差值（follow－up mean 4 weeks；Better indicated by lower values）

治疗结束后6个月便秘评分差值（follow－up mean 4 weeks；Better indicated by lower values）

治疗1周满意度评价（follow－up mean 4 weeks；Better indicated by lower values）

治疗2周满意度评价（follow－up mean 4 weeks；Better indicated by lower values）

| No of studies | Quality assessment | | | | | | No of patients | | Summary of findings | | Quality | Importance |
	Design	Limitations	Inconsistency	Indirectness	Imprecision	Other considerations	电针 VS 电针	control	Relative (95% CI)	Effect Absolute		
1	randomised trials	no serious limitations	no serious inconsistency	serious[3]	no serious imprecision	reporting bias[1]	30	30	–	SMD 0.08 higher (0.43 lower to 0.59 higher)	LOW	NOT IMPORTANT
1	randomised trials	no serious limitations	no serious inconsistency	serious[3]	no serious imprecision	reporting bias[1]	22	19	–	SMD 0.84 higher (0.2 to 1.49 higher)	LOW	NOT IMPORTANT
1	randomised trials	no serious limitations	no serious inconsistency	serious[3]	no serious imprecision	reporting bias[1]	22	19	–	SMD 0.62 higher (0.01 lower to 1.25 higher)	LOW	NOT IMPORTANT
1	randomised trials	no serious limitations	no serious inconsistency	serious[3]	no serious imprecision	reporting bias[1]	22	19	–	SMD 0.32 higher (0.3 lower to 0.93 higher)	LOW	NOT IMPORTANT
1	randomised trials	no serious limitations	no serious inconsistency	serious[3]	no serious imprecision	reporting bias[1]	48	23	–	SMD 0.55 lower (1.06 to 0.05 lower)	LOW	CRITICAL
1	randomised trials	no serious limitations	no serious inconsistency	serious[3]	no serious imprecision	reporting bias[1]	48	23	–	SMD 0.33 lower (0.83 lower to 0.17 higher)	LOW	CRITICAL

No of studies	Design	Quality assessment					No of patients		Summary of findings		Quality	Importance
		Limitations	Inconsistency	Indirectness	Imprecision	Other considerations	电针 VS 电针	control	Relative (95% CI)	Effect Absolute		
治疗 3 周满意度评价（follow－up mean 4 weeks；Better indicated by lower values）												
1	randomised trials	no serious limitations	no serious inconsistency	serious[3]	no serious imprecision	reporting bias[1]	48	23	-	SMD 0.59 lower（1.09 to 0.08 lower）	LOW	CRITICAL
治疗 4 周满意度评价（follow－up mean 4 weeks；Better indicated by lower values）												
1	randomised trials	no serious limitations	no serious inconsistency	serious[3]	no serious imprecision	reporting bias[1]	48	23	-	SMD 0.91 lower（1.43 to 0.39 lower）	LOW	CRITICAL
治疗前后焦虑自评量表 SAS 差值（follow－up mean 4 weeks；Better indicated by lower values）												
1	randomised trials	no serious limitations	no serious inconsistency	serious[3]	no serious imprecision	reporting bias[3]	30	30	-	SMD 0.29 lower（0.8 lower to 0.22 higher）	LOW	NOT IMPORTANT
治疗前后抑郁自评量表 SDS 差值（follow－up mean 4 weeks；Better indicated by lower values）												
1	randomised trials	no serious limitations	no serious inconsistency	serious[3]	no serious imprecision	reporting bias[1]	30	30	-	SMD 0.14 higher（0.37 lower to 0.65 higher）	LOW	NOT IMPORTANT
治疗前后症状自评量表 SCL－90 阳性项目数差值（follow－up mean 4 weeks；Better indicated by lower values）												
1	randomised trials	no serious limitations	no serious inconsistency	serious[3]	no serious imprecision	reporting bias[1]	30	30	-	SMD 0.1 higher（0.41 lower to 0.6 higher）	LOW	IMPORTANT
总有效率												
2	no methodology chosen	-	-	-	-	none	56/60 （93.3%）	47/60 （78.3%）	RR 1.18 （0.97 to 1.44）	141 more per 1000（from 23 fewer to 345 more）	-	-
								78.3%		141 more per 1000（from 23 fewer to 345 more）	-	-

No of studies	Quality assessment						Summary of findings					
	Design	Limitations	Inconsistency	Indirectness	Imprecision	Other considerations	No of patients		Effect		Quality	Importance
							电针 VS 电针	control	Relative (95% CI)	Absolute		
总有效率 - 深刺天枢 VS 浅刺天枢 (follow - up mean 4 weeks; revman)												
1	randomised trials	no serious limitations	no serious inconsistency	serious[3]	no serious imprecision	reporting bias[1]	29/30 (96.7%)	22/30 (73.3%) / 73.3%	RR 1.32 (1.05 to 1.65)	235 more per 1000 (from 37 more to 477 more) / 235 more per 1000 (from 37 more to 476 more)	LOW	CRITICAL
总有效率 - 深刺天枢 VS 浅刺天枢 (follow - up mean 4 weeks; revman)												
1	randomised trials	no serious limitations	no serious inconsistency	serious[3]	no serious imprecision	reporting bias[3]	27/30 (90%)	25/30 (83.3%) / 83.3%	RR 1.08 (0.88 to 1.32)	67 more per 1000 (from 100 fewer to 267 more) / 67 more per 1000 (from 100 fewer to 267 more)	LOW	CRITICAL
治疗前后结肠传输时间差值 (follow - up mean 4 weeks; Better indicated by lower values)												
1	randomised trials	no serious limitations	no serious inconsistency	no serious directness	no serious imprecision	reporting bias[1]	8	21	-	SMD 0.31 higher (0.51 lower to 1.12 higher)	MODERATE	NOT IMPORTANT
治疗1周排便费力程度评分差值 (follow - up mean 4 weeks; Better indicated by lower values)												
2	randomised trials	no serious limitations	no serious inconsistency	serious[3]	no serious imprecision	none	78	53	-	SMD 0.23 higher (0.28 lower to 0.74 higher)	MODERATE	NOT IMPORTANT
治疗1周排便费力程度评分差值 - 深刺天枢 VS 浅刺天枢 (Better indicated by lower values)												
2	no methodology chosen	-	-	-	-	none	78	53	-	SMD 0.23 higher (0.28 lower to 0.74 higher)	-	NOT IMPORTANT
治疗2周排便费力程度评分差值 (follow - up mean 4 weeks; Better indicated by lower values)												
2	randomised trials	no serious limitations	no serious inconsistency	serious[3]	no serious imprecision	none	78	53	-	SMD 0.15 higher (0.2 lower to 0.51 higher)	MODERATE	NOT IMPORTANT

续表

No of studies	Quality assessment						No of patients		Summary of findings		Quality	Importance
	Design	Limitations	Inconsistency	Indirectness	Imprecision	Other considerations	电针 VS 电针	control	Effect			
									Relative (95% CI)	Absolute		
治疗 4 周结束排便费力程度差值（Better indicated by lower values）												
3	no methodology chosen	-	-	-	-	none	108	83	-	SMD 0.36 higher (0.07 to 0.66 higher)	-	-
治疗 4 周结束排便费力程度差值 － 深刺天枢 VS 浅刺天枢（follow－up mean 4 weeks；Better indicated by lower values）												
2	randomised trials	no serious limitations	no serious inconsistency	serious[3]	no serious imprecision	none	78	53	-	SMD 0.51 higher (0.15 to 0.87 higher)	MODERATE	NOT IMPORTANT
治疗 4 周结束排便费力程度差值 － 低频电针 VS 高频电针（follow－up mean 4 weeks；Better indicated by lower values）												
1	randomised trials	no serious limitations	no serious inconsistency	serious[3]	no serious imprecision	reporting bias[1]	30	30	-	SMD 0.06 higher (0.44 lower to 0.57 higher)	LOW	NOT IMPORTANT
治疗结束 12 周排便力程度评分差值（follow－up mean 4 weeks；Better indicated by lower values）												
2	randomised trials	no serious limitations	no serious inconsistency	serious[3]	no serious imprecision	none	52	49	-	SMD 1.01 higher (0.59 to 1.42 higher)	MODERATE	NOT IMPORTANT
治疗结束 24 周排便力程度评分差值（follow－up mean 4 months；Better indicated by lower values）												
2	randomised trials	no serious limitations	no serious inconsistency	serious[3]	no serious imprecision	none	52	49	-	SMD 0.87 higher (0.46 to 1.28 higher)	MODERATE	NOT IMPORTANT
治疗 4 周结束后排便不尽感差值（Better indicated by lower values）												
3	no methodology chosen	-	-	-	-	none	108	83	-	SMD 0.37 higher (0.18 lower to 0.93 higher)	-	-

No of studies	Design	\<Quality assessment\> Limitations	Inconsistency	Indirectness	Imprecision	Other considerations	No of patients 电针 VS 电针	control	Effect Relative (95% CI)	Effect Absolute	Quality	Importance
治疗 4 周结束后排便不尽感差值 - 深刺天枢 VS 浅刺天枢(follow - up mean 4 weeks; Better indicated by lower values)												
2	randomised trials	no serious limitations	serious[2]	serious[3]	no serious imprecision	none	78	53	–	SMD 0.56 higher (0.19 lower to 1.31 higher)	LOW	NOT IMPORTANT
治疗 4 周结束后排便不尽感差值 - 低频电针 VS 高频电针(follow - up mean 4 weeks; Better indicated by lower values)												
1	randomised trials	no serious limitations	no serious inconsistency	serious[3]	no serious imprecision	reporting bias[1]	30	30	–	SMD 0.01 higher (0.5 lower to 0.52 higher)	LOW	NOT IMPORTANT
治疗结束后 12 周排便不尽感差值(follow - up mean 4 weeks; Better indicated by lower values)												
1	randomised trials	no serious limitations	no serious inconsistency	serious[3]	no serious imprecision	reporting bias[1]	30	30	–	SMD 1.31 higher (0.74 to 1.87 higher)	LOW	NOT IMPORTANT
治疗结束后 24 周排便不尽感差值(follow - up mean 4 weeks; Better indicated by lower values)												
1	randomised trials	no serious limitations	no serious inconsistency	serious[3]	no serious imprecision	reporting bias[1]	30	30	–	SMD 1.38 higher (0.82 to 1.95 higher)	LOW	NOT IMPORTANT
治疗 4 周大便质地差值(follow - up mean 4 weeks; Better indicated by lower values)												
2	randomised trials	no serious limitations	no serious inconsistency	serious[3]	no serious imprecision	none	78	53	–	SMD 0.28 higher (0.08 lower to 0.63 higher)	MODERATE	NOT IMPORTANT
治疗后 24 周大便质地差值(follow - up mean 4 weeks; Better indicated by lower values)												
1	randomised trials	no serious limitations	no serious inconsistency	serious[3]	no serious imprecision	reporting bias[1]	30	30	–	SMD 0.57 higher (0.06 to 1.09 higher)	LOW	NOT IMPORTANT

续表

No of studies	Quality assessment						No of patients 电针 VS 电针		Summary of findings		Quality	Importance
	Design	Limitations	Inconsistency	Indirectness	Imprecision	Other considerations		control	Effect			
									Relative (95% CI)	Absolute		
治疗4周结束排便频率评分差值（follow－up mean 4 weeks；Better indicated by lower values）												
1	randomised trials	no serious limitations	no serious inconsistency	no serious indirectness	no serious imprecision	reporting bias[1]	30	30	–	SMD 0.42 higher (0.09 lower to 0.94 higher)	MODERATE	NOT IMPORTANT
治疗结束后12周排便频率评分差值（follow－up mean 4 weeks；Better indicated by lower values）												
1	randomised trials	no serious limitations	no serious inconsistency	no serious indirectness	no serious imprecision	reporting bias[1]	22	19	–	SMD 1.04 higher (0.38 to 1.69 higher)	MODERATE	NOT IMPORTANT
治疗结束后6个月排便频率评分差值（follow－up mean 4 weeks；Better indicated by lower values）												
1	randomised trials	no serious limitations	no serious inconsistency	no serious indirectness	no serious imprecision	reporting bias[1]	22	19	–	SMD 0.87 higher (0.22 to 1.51 higher)	MODERATE	NOT IMPORTANT

1 只有一篇文章纳入。
2 异质性。
3 主观指标。

Author（s）:

Date: 2011 – 06 – 06

Question: 电针 VS 药物 for 慢性便秘

Settings:

Bibliography: 针灸 for 慢性便秘. Cochrane Database of Systematic Reviews [Year], Issue [Issue].

No of studies	Quality assessment						No of patients		Effect		Quality	Importance
	Design	Limitations	Inconsistency	Indirectness	Imprecision	Other considerations	电针 VS 药物	control	Relative (95% CI)	Absolute		
治疗 4 周排便次数差值（Better indicated by lower values）												
3	no methodology chosen	-	-	-	-	none	218	126	-	SMD 0.13 lower（0.58 lower to 0.32 higher）	-	NOT IMPORTANT
治疗 4 周排便次数差值 – 深刺天枢 VS 药物（follow – up mean 4 weeks; Better indicated by lower values）												
3	randomised trials	no serious limitations	no serious inconsistency	no serious indirectness	no serious imprecision	none	145	63	-	SMD 0.24 higher（0.05 lower to 0.54 higher）	HIGH	NOT IMPORTANT
治疗 4 周排便次数差值 – 常规刺天枢 VS 药物（follow – up mean 4 weeks; Better indicated by lower values）												
1	randomised trials	no serious limitations	no serious inconsistency	no serious indirectness	no serious imprecision	reporting bias[1]	28	21	-	SMD 0.16 lower（0.73 lower to 0.41 higher）	MODERATE	NOT IMPORTANT
治疗 4 周排便次数差值 – 浅刺天枢 VS 药物（follow – up mean 4 weeks; Better indicated by lower values）												
2	randomised trials	no serious limitations	serious[2]	no serious indirectness	no serious imprecision	reporting bias[3]	45	42	-	SMD 0.73 lower（1.85 lower to 0.39 higher）	LOW	NOT IMPORTANT
治疗 2 周总有效率（follow – up mean 4 weeks; revman）												
1	randomised trials	no serious limitations	no serious inconsistency	serious[4]	no serious imprecision	reporting bias[1]	23/30（76.7%）	6/30（20%）; 20%	RR 3.83（1.82 to 8.05）	566 more per 1000（from 164 more to 1410 more）; 566 more per 1000（from 164 more to 1410 more）	LOW	CRITICAL

续表

No of studies	Design	Limitations	Inconsistency	Indirectness	Imprecision	Other considerations	电针 VS 药物	control	Relative (95% CI)	Absolute	Quality	Importance
			Quality assessment				No of patients		Effect			
治疗 2 周 CCS 评分差值（follow – up mean 2 weeks; Better indicated by lower values）												
1	randomised trials	no serious limitations	no serious inconsistency	serious[4]	no serious imprecision	reporting bias[1]	30	30	–	SMD 0.61 higher (0.09 to 1.13 higher)	LOW	NOT IMPORTANT
治疗 2 周结束后 6 个月总有效率（follow – up mean 26 weeks; revman）												
1	randomised trials	no serious limitations	no serious inconsistency	serious[4]	no serious imprecision	reporting bias[1]	13/22 (59.1%)	1/19 (5.3%) / 5.3%	RR 11.23 (1.61 to 78.06)	538 more per 1000 (from 32 more to 4056 more) / 542 more per 1000 (from 32 more to 4084 more)	LOW	CRITICAL
治疗 2 周结束后 6 个月 CCS 评分差值（follow – up mean 26 weeks; Better indicated by lower values）												
1	randomised trials	no serious limitations	no serious inconsistency	serious[4]	no serious imprecision	reporting bias[1]	22	19	–	SMD 1.31 higher (0.63 to 2 higher)	LOW	NOT IMPORTANT
治疗 2 周 CTT 差值（follow – up mean 2 weeks; Better indicated by lower values）												
1	randomised trials	no serious limitations	no serious inconsistency	no serious indirectness	no serious imprecision	reporting bias[1]	30	30	–	SMD 1.17 higher (0.62 to 1.72 higher)	MODERATE	IMPORTANT
治疗 4 周 CCS 评分差值（Better indicated by lower values）												
4	no methodology chosen	-	-	-	-	none	259	168	–	SMD 0.61 higher (0.13 to 1.08 higher)	-	NOT IMPORTANT
治疗 4 周 CCS 评分差值 – 深刺天枢 VS 药物（follow – up mean 4 weeks; Better indicated by lower values）												
4	randomised trials	no serious limitations	serious[2]	serious[4]	no serious imprecision	none	167	84	–	SMD 0.94 higher (0.38 to 1.51 higher)	LOW	NOT IMPORTANT

No of studies	Design	Limitations	Inconsistency	Indirectness	Imprecision	Other considerations	No of patients 电针 VS 药物	control	Relative (95% CI)	Effect Absolute	Quality	Importance
治疗 4 周 CCS 评分差值 – 常规刺天枢 VS 药物（follow – up mean 4 weeks; Better indicated by lower values）												
2	randomised trials	no serious limitations	no serious inconsistency	serious[4]	no serious imprecision	none	47	42	-	SMD 0.17 lower (0.84 lower to 0.51 higher)	MODERATE	NOT IMPORTANT
治疗 4 周 CCS 评分差值 – 浅刺天枢 VS 药物（follow – up mean 4 weeks; Better indicated by lower values）												
2	randomised trials	no serious limitations	serious[2]	serious[4]	no serious imprecision	none	45	42	-	SMD 0.71 higher (0.22 lower to 1.64 higher)	LOW	NOT IMPORTANT
治疗 4 周结束后 12 周 CCS 评分差值（Better indicated by lower values）												
1	no methodology chosen	-	-	-	-	none	41	42	-	SMD 0.41 higher (0.2 lower to 1.02 higher)	-	CRITICAL
治疗 4 周结束后 12 周 CCS 评分差值 – 深刺天枢 VS 药物（follow – up mean 16 weeks; Better indicated by lower values）												
1	randomised trials	no serious limitations	no serious inconsistency	serious[4]	serious[5]	reporting bias[1]	22	21	-	SMD 0.72 higher (0.1 to 1.34 higher)	VERY LOW	NOT IMPORTANT
治疗 4 周结束后 12 周 CCS 评分差值 – 常规刺天枢 VS 药物（follow – up mean 16 weeks; Better indicated by lower values）												
1	randomised trials	no serious limitations	no serious inconsistency	serious[4]	serious[5]	reporting bias[1]	19	21	-	SMD 0.1 higher (0.52 lower to 0.72 higher)	VERY LOW	NOT IMPORTANT
治疗 4 周结束后 6 个月 CCS 评分差值（Better indicated by lower values）												
1	no methodology chosen	-	-	-	-	none	41	42	-	SMD 0.21 higher (0.22 lower to 0.64 higher)	-	NOT IMPORTANT
治疗 4 周结束后 6 个月 CCS 评分差值 – 深刺天枢 VS 药物（follow – up mean 28 weeks; Better indicated by lower values）												
1	randomised trials	no serious limitations	no serious inconsistency	serious[4]	serious[5]	reporting bias[1]	22	21	-	SMD 0.36 higher (0.24 lower to 0.97 higher)	VERY LOW	NOT IMPORTANT

续表

No of studies	Quality assessment						No of patients		Summary of findings		Quality	Importance
	Design	Limitations	Inconsistency	Indirectness	Imprecision	Other considerations	电针 VS 药物	control	Effect			
									Relative (95% CI)	Absolute		
治疗4周结束后6个月 CCS评分差值 - 常规刺天枢 VS 药物（follow-up mean 28 weeks; Better indicated by lower values）												
1	randomised trials	no serious limitations	no serious inconsistency	serious[4]	serious[5]	reporting bias[1]	19	21	-	SMD 0.05 higher (0.57 lower to 0.67 higher)	VERY LOW	NOT IMPORTANT
治疗4周结束后4周排便频率评分差值（Better indicated by lower values）												
1	no methodology chosen	-	-	-	-	none	41	42	-	SMD 0.12 lower (1.54 lower to 1.3 higher)	-	-
治疗4周结束后4周排便频率评分差值 - 深刺天枢 VS 药物（follow-up mean 8 weeks; Better indicated by lower values）												
1	randomised trials	no serious limitations	no serious inconsistency	no serious indirectness	serious[5]	reporting bias[1]	22	21	-	SMD 0.6 higher (0.02 lower to 1.21 higher)	LOW	NOT IMPORTANT
治疗4周结束后4周排便频率评分差值 - 常规刺天枢 VS 药物（follow-up mean 8 weeks; Better indicated by lower values）												
1	randomised trials	no serious limitations	no serious inconsistency	no serious indirectness	serious[5]	reporting bias[1]	19	21	-	SMD 0.85 lower (1.5 to 0.2 lower)	LOW	NOT IMPORTANT
治疗4周结束后12周排便频率评分差值（Better indicated by lower values）												
1	no methodology chosen	-	-	-	-	none	41	42	-	SMD 0.15 lower (1.16 lower to 0.87 higher)	-	-
治疗4周结束后12周排便频率评分差值 - 深刺天枢 VS 药物（follow-up mean 16 weeks; Better indicated by lower values）												
1	randomised trials	no serious limitations	no serious inconsistency	no serious indirectness	serious[5]	reporting bias[1]	22	21	-	SMD 0.37 higher (0.24 lower to 0.97 higher)	LOW	NOT IMPORTANT
治疗4周结束后12周排便频率评分差值 - 常规刺天枢 VS 药物（follow-up mean 16 weeks; Better indicated by lower values）												
1	randomised trials	no serious limitations	no serious inconsistency	no serious indirectness	serious[5]	reporting bias[1]	19	21	-	SMD 0.67 lower (1.31 to 0.03 lower)	LOW	NOT IMPORTANT

续表

No of studies	Quality assessment						No of patients		Summary of findings		Quality	Importance
	Design	Limitations	Inconsistency	Indirectness	Imprecision	Other considerations	电针 VS 药物	control	Relative (95% CI)	Effect — Absolute		
治疗4周结束后6个月排便频率评分差值（Better indicated by lower values）												
1	no methodology chosen	-	-	-	-	none	41	42	-	SMD 0.14 lower（0.97 lower to 0.68 higher）	-	-
治疗4周结束后6个月排便频率评分差值 - 深刺天枢 VS 药物（follow-up mean 28 weeks; Better indicated by lower values）												
1	randomised trials	no serious limitations	no serious consistency	no serious indirectness	serious[5]	reporting bias[1]	22	21	-	SMD 0.27 higher（0.33 lower to 0.87 higher）	LOW	NOT IMPORTANT
治疗4周结束后6个月排便频率评分差值 - 深刺天枢 VS 药物（follow-up mean 28 weeks; Better indicated by lower values）												
1	randomised trials	no serious limitations	no serious consistency	no serious indirectness	serious[5]	reporting bias[1]	22	21	-	SMD 0.27 higher（0.33 lower to 0.87 higher）	LOW	NOT IMPORTANT
治疗4周后排便频率评分差值（Better indicated by lower values）												
1	no methodology chosen	-	-	-	-	none	87	42	-	SMD 0.03 higher（0.35 lower to 0.4 higher）	-	-
治疗4周后排便频率评分差值 - 深刺天枢 VS 药物（follow-up mean 4 weeks; Better indicated by lower values）												
1	randomised trials	no serious limitations	no serious consistency	no serious indirectness	no serious imprecision	reporting bias[1]	59	21	-	SMD 0.17 higher（0.33 lower to 0.67 higher）	MODERATE	NOT IMPORTANT
治疗4周后排便频率评分差值 - 常规刺天枢 VS 药物（follow-up mean 4 weeks; Better indicated by lower values）												
1	randomised trials	no serious limitations	no serious consistency	no serious indirectness	no serious imprecision	reporting bias[1]	28	21	-	SMD 0.15 lower（0.72 lower to 0.42 higher）	MODERATE	NOT IMPORTANT
治疗4周后排便费力程度评分差值（Better indicated by lower values）												
2	no methodology chosen	-	-	-	-	none	158	90	-	SMD 0.59 higher（0.06 lower to 1.24 higher）	-	-

续表

No of studies	Quality assessment						No of patients		Summary of findings			
	Design	Limitations	Inconsistency	Indirectness	Imprecision	Other considerations	电针 VS 药物	control	Effect		Quality	Importance
									Relative (95% CI)	Absolute		
治疗 4 周排便费力程度评分差值 – 深刺天枢 VS 药物 (follow – up mean 4 weeks; Better indicated by lower values)												
2	randomised trials	no serious limitations	serious[2]	serious[4]	no serious imprecision	reporting bias[3]	107	45	–	SMD 0.73 higher (0.48 lower to 1.95 higher)	VERY LOW	NOT IMPORTANT
治疗 4 周排便费力程度评分差值 – 深刺天枢 VS 药物 (follow – up mean 4 weeks; Better indicated by lower values)												
2	randomised trials	no serious limitations	serious[2]	serious[4]	no serious imprecision	reporting bias[3]	107	45	–	SMD 0.73 higher (0.48 lower to 1.95 higher)	VERY LOW	NOT IMPORTANT
治疗 4 周排便费力程度评分差值 – 浅刺天枢 VS 药物 (follow – up mean 4 weeks; Better indicated by lower values)												
1	randomised trials	no serious limitations	no serious inconsistency	serious[4]	no serious imprecision	reporting bias[1]	23	24	–	SMD 0.92 higher (0.32 to 1.53 higher)	LOW	NOT IMPORTANT
治疗 4 周结束后 4 周排便费力程度评分差值 (Better indicated by lower values)												
1	no methodology chosen	–	–	–	–	none	41	42	–	SMD 0.2 higher (0.88 lower to 1.29 higher)	–	–
治疗 4 周结束后 4 周排便费力程度评分差值 – 深刺天枢 VS 药物 (follow – up mean 8 weeks; Better indicated by lower values)												
1	randomised trials	no serious limitations	no serious inconsistency	serious[4]	no serious imprecision	reporting bias[1]	22	21	–	SMD 0.75 higher (0.13 to 1.37 higher)	LOW	NOT IMPORTANT
治疗 4 周结束后 4 周排便费力程度评分差值 – 常规刺天枢 VS 药物 (follow – up mean 8 weeks; Better indicated by lower values)												
1	randomised trials	no serious limitations	no serious inconsistency	serious[4]	no serious imprecision	reporting bias[1]	19	21	–	SMD 0.35 lower (0.98 lower to 0.27 higher)	LOW	NOT IMPORTANT
治疗 4 周结束后 12 周排便费力程度评分差值 (follow – up mean 4 weeks; Better indicated by lower values)												
1	randomised trials	no serious limitations	no serious inconsistency	serious[4]	no serious imprecision	reporting bias[1]	41	42	–	SMD 0.29 lower (1.46 lower to 0.87 higher)	LOW	NOT IMPORTANT

续表

No of studies	Quality assessment						No of patients		Summary of findings		Quality	Importance
	Design	Limitations	Inconsistency	Indirectness	Imprecision	Other considerations	电针 VS 药物	control	Effect			
									Relative (95% CI)	Absolute		
治疗 4 周结束后 12 周排便费力程度评分差值 – 深刺天枢 VS 药物（follow – up mean 16 weeks; Better indicated by lower values）												
1	randomised trials	no serious limitations	no serious inconsistency	serious[4]	no serious imprecision	reporting bias[1]	22	21	–	SMD 0.29 higher (0.31 lower to 0.89 higher)	LOW	NOT IMPORTANT
治疗 4 周结束后 12 周排便费力程度评分差值 – 常规刺天枢 VS 药物（follow – up mean 16 weeks; Better indicated by lower values）												
1	randomised trials	no serious limitations	no serious inconsistency	serious[5]	no serious imprecision	reporting bias[1]	19	21	–	SMD 0.89 lower (1.55 to 0.24 lower)	LOW	NOT IMPORTANT
治疗 4 周结束后 6 个月排便费力程度评分差值（Better indicated by lower values）												
1	no methodology chosen	–	–	–	–	none	41	42	–	SMD 0 higher (0.65 lower to 0.64 higher)	–	–
治疗 4 周结束后 6 个月排便费力程度评分差值 – 深刺天枢 VS 药物（follow – up mean 28 weeks; Better indicated by lower values）												
1	randomised trials	no serious limitations	no serious inconsistency	serious[4]	no serious imprecision	reporting bias[1]	22	21	–	SMD 0.32 higher (0.28 lower to 0.92 higher)	LOW	NOT IMPORTANT
治疗 4 周结束后 6 个月排便费力程度评分差值 – 常规刺天枢 VS 药物（follow – up mean 28 weeks; Better indicated by lower values）												
1	randomised trials	no serious limitations	no serious inconsistency	serious[4]	no serious imprecision	reporting bias[1]	19	21	–	SMD 0.34 lower (0.97 lower to 0.28 higher)	LOW	NOT IMPORTANT
治疗 4 周排便时间评分差值（Better indicated by lower values）												
1	no methodology chosen	–	–	–	–	none	87	42	–	SMD 0.22 higher (0.15 lower to 0.6 higher)	–	–
治疗 4 周排便时间评分差值 – 深刺天枢 VS 药物（follow – up mean 4 weeks; Better indicated by lower values）												
1	randomised trials	no serious limitations	no serious inconsistency	no serious indirectness	no serious imprecision	reporting bias[1]	59	21	–	SMD 0.39 higher (0.12 lower to 0.89 higher)	MODERATE	NOT IMPORTANT

续表

No of studies	Design	Limitations	Inconsistency	Indirectness	Imprecision	Other considerations	电针 VS 药物	control	Relative (95% CI)	Absolute	Quality	Importance
治疗4周排便时间评分差值 - 常规刺天枢 VS 药物（follow – up mean 4 weeks；Better indicated by lower values）												
1	randomised trials	no serious limitations	no serious inconsistency	no serious indirectness	no serious imprecision	reporting bias[1]	28	21	-	SMD 0.02 higher (0.55 lower to 0.58 higher)	MODERATE	NOT IMPORTANT
治疗4周结束后4周排便时间评分差值（Better indicated by lower values）												
1	no methodology chosen	-	-	-	-	none	41	42	-	SMD 0.22 higher (0.25 lower to 0.69 higher)	-	-
治疗4周排便时间评分差值 - 深刺天枢 VS 药物（follow – up mean 8 weeks；Better indicated by lower values）												
1	randomised trials	no serious limitations	no serious inconsistency	no serious indirectness	no serious imprecision	reporting bias[1]	22	21	-	SMD 0.46 higher (0.15 lower to 1.07 higher)	MODERATE	NOT IMPORTANT
治疗4周排便时间评分差值 - 常规刺天枢 VS 药物（follow – up mean 8 weeks；Better indicated by lower values）												
1	randomised trials	no serious limitations	no serious inconsistency	no serious indirectness	no serious imprecision	reporting bias[1]	19	21	-	SMD 0.02 lower (0.64 lower to 0.6 higher)	MODERATE	NOT IMPORTANT
治疗4周结束后12周排便时间评分差值（Better indicated by lower values）												
1	no methodology chosen	-	-	-	-	none	41	42	-	SMD 0.12 higher (0.31 lower to 0.56 higher)	-	-
治疗4周结束后12周排便时间评分差值 - 深刺天枢 VS 药物（follow – up mean 16 weeks；Better indicated by lower values）												
1	randomised trials	no serious limitations	no serious inconsistency	no serious indirectness	no serious imprecision	reporting bias[1]	22	21	-	SMD 0.27 higher (0.33 lower to 0.87 higher)	MODERATE	NOT IMPORTANT
治疗4周结束后12周排便时间评分差值 - 常规刺天枢 VS 药物（follow – up mean 16 weeks；Better indicated by lower values）												
1	randomised trials	no serious limitations	no serious inconsistency	no serious indirectness	no serious imprecision	reporting bias[1]	19	21	-	SMD 0.03 lower (0.65 lower to 0.59 higher)	MODERATE	NOT IMPORTANT

| No of studies | Design | Limitations | Inconsistency | Indirectness | Imprecision | Other considerations | No of patients | | Relative (95% CI) | Effect | Quality | Importance |
							电针 VS 药物	control		Absolute		
治疗 4 周结束后 6 个月排便时间评分差值（Better indicated by lower values）												
1	no methodology chosen	-	-	-	-	none	41	42	-	SMD 0.02 lower (0.45 lower to 0.41 higher)	-	-
治疗 4 周结束后 6 个月排便时间评分差值 – 深刺天枢 VS 药物（follow – up mean 28 weeks；Better indicated by lower values）												
1	randomised trials	no serious limitations	no serious inconsistency	no serious indirectness	no serious imprecision	reporting bias[1]	22	21	-	SMD 0.02 higher (0.58 lower to 0.62 higher)	MODERATE	NOT IMPORTANT
治疗 4 周结束后 6 个月排便时间评分差值 – 常规刺天枢 VS 药物（follow – up mean 28 weeks；Better indicated by lower values）												
1	randomised trials	no serious limitations	no serious inconsistency	no serious indirectness	no serious imprecision	reporting bias[1]	19	21	-	SMD 0.07 lower (0.69 lower to 0.55 higher)	MODERATE	NOT IMPORTANT
治疗 4 周后 CTT 时间差值（Better indicated by lower values）												
1	no methodology chosen	-	-	-	-	none	87	42	-	SMD 0.1 higher (0.27 lower to 0.48 higher)	-	-
治疗 4 周后 CTT 时间差值 – 深刺天枢 VS 药物（follow – up mean 4 days；Better indicated by lower values）												
1	randomised trials	no serious limitations	no serious inconsistency	no serious indirectness	no serious imprecision	reporting bias[1]	59	21	-	SMD 0.15 higher (0.34 lower to 0.65 higher)	MODERATE	IMPORTANT
治疗 4 周后 CTT 时间差值 – 常规刺天枢 VS 药物（follow – up mean 4 weeks；Better indicated by lower values）												
1	randomised trials	no serious limitations	no serious inconsistency	no serious indirectness	no serious imprecision	reporting bias[1]	28	21	-	SMD 0.04 higher (0.53 lower to 0.6 higher)	MODERATE	IMPORTANT
首次排便时间（Better indicated by lower values）												
1	no methodology chosen	-	-	-	-	none	87	42	-	SMD 0.29 lower (1.32 lower to 0.75 higher)	-	-

续表

No of studies	Design	Quality assessment					No of patients		Summary of findings		Quality	Importance
		Limitations	Inconsistency	Indirectness	Imprecision	Other considerations	电针 VS 药物	control	Relative (95% CI)	Effect Absolute		
首次排便时间 – 深刺天枢 VS 药物 (follow – up mean 4 weeks; Better indicated by lower values)												
1	randomised trials	no serious limitations	no serious inconsistency	no serious indirectness	no serious imprecision	reporting bias[1]	59	21	–	SMD 0.81 lower (1.32 to 0.29 lower)	MODERATE	NOT IMPORTANT
首次排便时间 – 常规刺天枢 VS 药物 (follow – up mean 4 weeks; Better indicated by lower values)												
1	randomised trials	no serious limitations	no serious inconsistency	no serious indirectness	no serious imprecision	reporting bias[1]	28	21	–	SMD 0.25 higher (0.32 lower to 0.82 higher)	MODERATE	NOT IMPORTANT
治疗 4 周结束后 4 周排便次数差值 (Better indicated by lower values)												
1	no methodology chosen	–	–	–	–	none	72	46	–	SMD 0.33 lower (1.66 lower to 0.99 higher)	–	–
治疗 4 周结束后 4 周排便次数差值 – 深刺天枢 VS 药物 (follow – up mean 8 weeks; Better indicated by lower values)												
1	randomised trials	no serious limitations	no serious inconsistency	no serious indirectness	no serious imprecision	reporting bias[1]	48	23	–	SMD 0.33 higher (0.17 lower to 0.83 higher)	MODERATE	NOT IMPORTANT
治疗 4 周结束后 4 周排便次数差值 – 浅刺天枢 VS 药物 (follow – up mean 8 weeks; Better indicated by lower values)												
1	randomised trials	no serious limitations	no serious inconsistency	no serious indirectness	no serious imprecision	reporting bias[1]	24	23	–	SMD 1.02 lower (1.63 to 0.41 lower)	MODERATE	NOT IMPORTANT
治疗 4 周结束后 12 周排便次数差值 (Better indicated by lower values)												
1	no methodology chosen	–	–	–	–	none	72	46	–	SMD 0 higher (0.89 lower to 0.89 higher)	–	–
治疗 4 周结束后 12 周排便次数差值 – 深刺天枢 VS 药物 (follow – up mean 16 weeks; Better indicated by lower values)												
1	randomised trials	no serious limitations	no serious inconsistency	no serious indirectness	no serious imprecision	reporting bias[1]	48	23	–	SMD 0.44 higher (0.06 lower to 0.94 higher)	MODERATE	NOT IMPORTANT

续表

No of studies	Quality assessment						No of patients		Summary of findings		Quality	Importance
	Design	Limitations	Inconsistency	Indirectness	Imprecision	Other considerations	电针 VS 药物	control	Effect			
									Relative (95% CI)	Absolute		
治疗 4 周结束后 12 周排便次数差值（follow – up mean 16 weeks；Better indicated by lower values）												
1	randomised trials	no serious limitations	no serious inconsistency	no serious indirectness	no serious imprecision	reporting bias[1]	24	23	–	SMD 0.47 lower（1.05 lower to 0.11 higher）	MODERATE	NOT IMPORTANT
治疗 4 周结束后 6 个月排便次数差值（Better indicated by lower values）												
1	no methodology chosen	–	–	–	–	none	72	46	–	SMD 0.17 higher（1.22 lower to 1.57 higher）		–
治疗 4 周结束后 6 个月排便次数差值 – 深刺天枢 VS 药物（follow – up mean 28 weeks；Better indicated by lower values）												
1	randomised trials	no serious limitations	no serious inconsistency	no serious indirectness	no serious imprecision	reporting bias[1]	48	23	–	SMD 0.88 higher（0.36 to 1.4 higher）	MODERATE	NOT IMPORTANT
治疗 4 周结束后 6 个月排便次数差值 – 浅刺天枢 VS 药物（follow – up mean 4 weeks；Better indicated by lower values）												
1	randomised trials	no serious limitations	no serious inconsistency	no serious indirectness	no serious imprecision	reporting bias[1]	24	23	–	SMD 0.54 lower（1.13 lower to 0.04 higher）	MODERATE	NOT IMPORTANT
治疗 4 周大便不尽感评分差值（follow – up mean 4 weeks；Better indicated by lower values）												
2	randomised trials	no serious limitations	no serious inconsistency	serious[4]	no serious imprecision	none	158	90	–	SMD 0.67 higher（0.3 to 1.03 higher）	MODERATE	NOT IMPORTANT
治疗 4 周大便不尽感评分差值 – 深刺天枢 VS 药物（follow – up mean 4 weeks；Better indicated by lower values）												
2	randomised trials	no serious limitations	no serious inconsistency	serious[4]	no serious imprecision	none	107	45	–	SMD 0.72 higher（0.11 to 1.33 higher）	MODERATE	NOT IMPORTANT
治疗 4 周大便不尽感评分差值 – 浅刺天枢 VS 药物（follow – up mean 4 weeks；Better indicated by lower values）												
1	randomised trials	no serious limitations	no serious inconsistency	serious[4]	no serious imprecision	reporting bias[1]	23	24	–	SMD 0.94 higher（0.33 to 1.54 higher）	LOW	NOT IMPORTANT

续表

No of studies	Quality assessment						No of patients		Summary of findings		Quality	Importance
	Design	Limitations	Inconsistency	Indirectness	Imprecision	Other considerations	电针 VS 药物	control	Effect			
									Relative (95% CI)	Absolute		
治疗 4 周大便不尽感评分差值 - 常规刺天枢 VS 药物（follow-up mean 4 weeks；Better indicated by lower values）												
1	randomised trials	no serious limitations	no serious inconsistency	serious[4]	no serious imprecision	reporting bias[1]	28	21	-	SMD 0.3 higher (0.27 lower to 0.87 higher)	LOW	NOT IMPORTANT
治疗 4 周大便质地评分差值（Better indicated by lower values）												
1	no methodology chosen	-	-	-	-	none	71	48	-	SMD 0.38 higher (0.01 to 0.76 higher)	-	-
治疗 4 周大便质地评分差值 - 深刺天枢 VS 药物（follow-up mean 4 weeks；Better indicated by lower values）												
1	randomised trials	no serious limitations	no serious inconsistency	serious[4]	no serious imprecision	reporting bias[1]	48	24	-	SMD 0.47 higher (0.02 lower to 0.97 higher)	LOW	NOT IMPORTANT
治疗 4 周大便质地评分差值 - 浅刺天枢 VS 药物（follow-up mean 4 weeks；Better indicated by lower values）												
1	randomised trials	no serious limitations	no serious inconsistency	serious[4]	no serious imprecision	reporting bias[1]	23	24	-	SMD 0.26 higher (0.32 lower to 0.83 higher)	LOW	NOT IMPORTANT
治疗 4 周满意度评分差值（Better indicated by lower values）												
1	no methodology chosen	-	-	-	-	none	71	48	-	SMD 1.75 lower (2.48 to 1.03 lower)	-	-
治疗 4 周满意度评分差值 - 深刺天枢 VS 药物（follow-up mean 4 weeks；Better indicated by lower values）												
1	randomised trials	no serious limitations	no serious inconsistency	serious[4]	no serious imprecision	reporting bias[1]	48	24	-	SMD 2.12 lower (2.72 to 1.51 lower)	LOW	CRITICAL
治疗 4 周满意度评分差值 - 浅刺天枢 VS 药物（follow-up mean 4 weeks；Better indicated by lower values）												
1	randomised trials	no serious limitations	no serious inconsistency	serious[4]	no serious imprecision	reporting bias[1]	23	24	-	SMD 1.37 lower (2.02 to 0.73 lower)	LOW	CRITICAL

1 只有一篇纳入文献。
2 异质性较大。
3 未来发表文献有可能逆转结果。
4 主观性指标。
5 样本量小。

Author（s）：

Date：2011 – 07 – 20

Question：手针 + 生物反馈 VS 生物反馈 for 慢性便秘

Settings：

Bibliography：

No of studies	Quality assessment						No of patients		Summary of findings			
	Design	Limitations	Inconsistency	Indirectness	Imprecision	Other considerations	手针 + 生物反馈	生物反馈 VS 生物反馈	Effect		Quality	Importance
									Relative (95% CI)	Absolute		
治疗 3 周结束每周大便次数差值（follow – up mean 3 weeks；Better indicated by lower values）												
1	observational studies	serious[1]	no serious inconsistency	no serious indirectness	serious[2]	reporting bias[3]	25	20	–	SMD 0.39 lower（0 to 0.2 higher）	VERY LOW	NOT IMPORTANT
治疗结束 1 月后大便次数差值（follow – up mean 7 weeks；Better indicated by lower values）												
1	observational studies	serious[1]	no serious inconsistency	no serious indirectness	serious[2]	reporting bias[3]	25	20	–	SMD 0.88 higher（0.27 to 1.5 higher）	VERY LOW	NOT IMPORTANT
治疗 3 周结束排便困难积分（follow – up mean 3 weeks；Better indicated by lower values）												
1	observational studies	serious[1]	no serious inconsistency	serious[4]	serious[2]	reporting bias[3]	25	20	–	SMD 0.21 lower（0.71 lower to 0.47 higher）	VERY LOW	NOT IMPORTANT
治疗结束 1 月后排便困难积分（follow – up mean 7 weeks；Better indicated by lower values）												
1	observational studies	serious[1]	no serious inconsistency	serious[4]	serious[2]	reporting bias[3]	25	20	–	SMD 0.79 higher（0.17 to 1.4 higher）	VERY LOW	NOT IMPORTANT
治疗 3 周结束大便性状积分差值（follow – up mean 3 weeks；Better indicated by lower values）												
1	observational studies	serious[1]	no serious inconsistency	serious[4]	serious[2]	reporting bias[3]	25	20	–	SMD 0.46 higher（0.14 lower to 1.06 higher）	VERY LOW	NOT IMPORTANT

续表

No of studies	Design	Limitations	Inconsistency	Indirectness	Imprecision	Other considerations	手针＋生物反馈 反馈	生物 VS 生物反馈	Relative (95% CI)	Absolute	Quality	Importance
							No of patients		Effect			
		Quality assessment							Summary of findings			

治疗 3 周结束肛门直肠测压各项指标差值（follow – up mean 3 weeks；Better indicated by lower values）

| 1 | observational studies | serious[1] | no serious inconsistency | no serious indirectness | serious[2] | reporting bias[3] | 25 | 20 | - | MD 0 higher（0 to 0 higher） | VERY LOW | NOT IMPORTANT |

治疗结束 1 月肛门直肠测压各指标差值（follow – up mean 7 weeks；Better indicated by lower values）

| 1 | observational studies | serious[1] | no serious inconsistency | no serious indirectness | serious[2] | reporting bias[3] | 25 | 20 | - | MD 0 higher（0 to 0 higher） | VERY LOW | NOT IMPORTANT |

治疗结束 1 月大便性状积分差值（follow – up mean 7 weeks；Better indicated by lower values）

| 1 | observational studies | serious[1] | no serious inconsistency | serious4 | serious[2] | reporting bias[3] | 25 | 20 | - | SMD 1.15 higher（0.52 to 1.79 higher） | VERY LOW | NOT IMPORTANT |

1 非随机对照。
2 样本量小。
3 只有一篇文献纳入。
4 主观指标。

Author (s):

Date: 2011 – 07 – 21

Question: 电针＋电脑中频治疗仪 VS 电脑中频治疗仪 for 慢性便秘

Settings:

Bibliography:

No of studies	Quality assessment						No of patients		Summary of findings		Quality	Importance
	Design	Limitations	Inconsistency	Indirectness	Imprecision	Other considerations	电针＋电脑中频治疗仪 VS 电脑中频治疗仪		Effect			
									Relative (95% CI)	Absolute		
显效率 (follow – up mean 2 weeks)												
1	observational studies	serious[1]	no serious inconsistency	serious[2]	no serious imprecision	reporting bias[3]	24/31 (77.4%)	18/30 (60%) 60%	18/30 (60%) 60%	174 more per 1000 (from 54 fewer to 498 more) 174 more per 1000 (from 54 fewer to 498 more)	VERY LOW	CRITICAL

1 非随机对照。

2 主观指标。

3 只有一篇文献纳入。

Author (s):

Date: 2011 – 08 – 01

Question: 两组穴位交替针刺 for 慢性功能性便秘

Settings:

Bibliography:

No of studies	Quality assessment						No of patients		Summary of findings		Quality	Importance
	Design	Limitations	Inconsistency	Indirectness	Imprecision	Other considerations	两组穴位交替针刺	control	Effect			
									Relative (95% CI)	Absolute		
生活质量积分 (follow – up mean 20 days; Better indicated by lower values)												
1	observational studies[1]	serious[2]	no serious inconsistency	serious[3]	no serious imprecision	reporting bias[4]	90	0	–	mean 0 higher (0 to 0 higher)	VERY LOW	IMPORTANT
症状积分 (follow – up mean 20 days; Better indicated by lower values)												
1	observational studies[1]	serious[2]	no serious inconsistency	serious[3]	no serious imprecision	reporting bias[4]	90	0	–	mean 0 higher (0 to 0 higher)	VERY LOW	NOT IMPORTANT
每次排便时间 (follow – up mean 20 days; Better indicated by lower values)												
1	observational studies[1]	serious[2]	no serious inconsistency	no serious indirectness	no serious imprecision	reporting bias[4]	90	0	–	mean 0 higher (0 to 0 higher)	VERY LOW	NOT IMPORTANT
治疗结束时有效率 (follow – up mean 20 days)												
1	observational studies[1]	serious[1]	no serious inconsistency	serious[3]	no serious imprecision	reporting bias[4]	72/90 (80%)	0/0 (0%)	RR 0 (0 to 0)	0 fewer per 1000 (from 0 fewer to 0 fewer)	VERY LOW	CRITICAL
治疗结束后1个月有效率 (follow – up mean 20 days)												
1	observational studies[1]	serious[1]	no serious inconsistency	serious[3]	no serious imprecision	reporting bias[4]	70/90 (77.8%)	0/0 (0%)	RR 0 (0 to 0)	0 fewer per 1000 (from 0 fewer to 0 fewer)	VERY LOW	CRITICAL

续表

治疗结束后 3 个月有效率（follow – up mean 20 days）

No of studies	Quality assessment						No of patients		Summary of findings		Quality	Importance
	Design	Limitations	Inconsistency	Indirectness	Imprecision	Other considerations	两组穴位交替针刺	control	Effect			
									Relative (95% CI)	Absolute		
1	observational studies[1]	serious[1]	no serious inconsistency	serious[3]	no serious imprecision	reporting bias[4]	62/90 (68.9%)	0/0 (0%)	RR 0 (0 to 0)	0 fewer per 1000 (from 0 fewer to 0 fewer)	VERY LOW	CRITICAL

1 Case Series.
2 观察性研究。
3 主观指标。
4 只有一篇文献纳入。

Author (s)：

Date：2011 – 08 – 02

Question：音频电疗 + 针刺 VS 针刺 for 老年习惯性便秘

Settings：

Bibliography：

有效率（follow – up mean 45 days）

No of studies	Quality assessment						No of patients		Summary of findings		Quality	Importance
	Design	Limitations	Inconsistency	Indirectness	Imprecision	Other considerations	音频电疗 + 针刺 VS 针刺	control	Effect			
									Relative (95% CI)	Absolute		
1	observational studies	serious[1]	no serious inconsistency	serious[2]	no serious imprecision	reporting bias[3]	88/90 (97.8%)	0%	OR 0 (0 to 0)	0 fewer per 1000 (from 0 fewer to 0 fewer)	VERY LOW	CRITICAL

1 Case – control.
2 主观性指标。
3 只纳入一篇文献。

Author（s）：

Date：2011 – 08 – 07

Question：针刺 + 腹部推拿 VS 五仁润肠丸 for 老年性虚证便秘

Settings：

Bibliography：

总有效率（follow – up mean 20 days）

No of studies	Quality assessment						No of patients		Summary of findings		Quality	Importance
	Design	Limitations	Inconsistency	Indirectness	Imprecision	Other considerations	针刺 + 腹部推拿 VS 五仁润肠丸		Effect			
							针刺 + 腹部推拿	五仁润肠丸	Relative (95% CI)	Absolute		
1	observational studies	serious[1]	no serious inconsistency	serious[2]	no serious imprecision	reporting bias[3]	29/30 (96.7%)	20/30 (66.7%)	RR 1.45 (1.12 to 1.88)	300 more per 1000 (from 80 more to 587 more)	VERY LOW	CRITICAL
								66.7%		300 more per 1000 (from 80 more to 587 more)		

1 假随机。

2 主观性指标。

3 只有一篇文献纳入。

Author (s)：

Date：2011 – 08 – 07

Question：水针 + 益气润肠汤 VS 麻仁丸 for 老年习惯性便秘

Settings：

Bibliography：

No of studies	Quality assessment						No of patients		Summary of findings			
	Design	Limitations	Inconsistency	Indirectness	Imprecision	Other considerations	水针 + 益气润肠汤	VS 麻仁丸	Effect		Quality	Importance
									Relative (95% CI)	Absolute		
有效率（follow – up mean 40 days）												
1	observational studies	serious[1]	no serious inconsistency	serious[2]	no serious imprecision	reporting bias[3]	196/196 (100%)	180/180 (100%) 100%	RR 1 (0.99 to 1.01)	0 fewer per 1000（from 10 fewer to 10 more）0 fewer per 1000（from 10 fewer to 10 more）	VERY LOW	CRITICAL
便秘消失时间（follow – up mean 40 days；Better indicated by lower values）												
1	observational studies	serious[1]	no serious inconsistency	no serious directness	no serious imprecision	reporting bias[3]	196	180	–	SMD 2.98 lower (3.28 to 2.69 lower)	VERY LOW	NOT IMPORTANT
便秘复发时间（follow – up mean 40 days；Better indicated by lower values）												
1	observational studies	serious[1]	no serious inconsistency	no serious directness	no serious imprecision	reporting bias[3]	196	180	–	SMD 44.68 higher (41.46 to 47.9 higher)	VERY LOW	NOT IMPORTANT

1 非随机对照试验。

2 主观性指标。

3 只有一篇文献纳入。

Author（s）：
Date：2011 – 08 – 08
Question：手针 for 糖尿病性便秘
Settings：
Bibliography：

总有效率（follow – up mean 34 days）

Quality assessment							Summary of findings					
							No of patients		Effect			
Quality assessment	Quality	assessment	Quality	assessment	Quality		手针	control	Relative (95% CI)	Absolute	Quality	Importance
1	observational studies[1]	serious[1]	no serious in-consistency	serious[2]	serious[3]	reporting bias[4]	28/30 (93.3%)	0/0 (0%)	RR 0 (0 to 0)	0 fewer per 1000 (from 0 fewer to 0 fewer)	VERY LOW	CRITICAL

1 Case Series.
2 主观性指标。
3 样本量小。
4 只有一篇文献纳入。

Author (s) :

Date: 2011 – 08 – 08

Question: 深刺天枢 for 结肠慢转运型便秘

Settings:

Bibliography:

No of studies	Quality assessment						No of patients		Summary of findings		Quality	Importance
	Design	Limitations	Inconsistency	Indirectness	Imprecision	Other considerations	深刺天枢	control	Effect			
									Relative (95% CI)	Absolute		
30 例的 CCS 积分 (follow – up mean 2 weeks; Better indicated by lower values)												
1	observational studies[1]	serious[1]	no serious inconsistency	serious[2]	serious[3]	reporting bias[4]	30	0	–	mean 0 higher (0 to 0 higher)	VERY LOW	NOT IMPORTANT
30 例的 CTT 结果 (follow – up mean 2 weeks; Better indicated by lower values)												
1	observational studies[1]	serious[1]	no serious inconsistency	no serious indirectness	serious[3]	reporting bias[4]	30	0	–	mean 0 higher (0 to 0 higher)	VERY LOW	IMPORTANT
30 例的 CCS 有效率 (follow – up mean 2 weeks)												
1	observational studies[1]	serious[1]	no serious inconsistency	serious[2]	serious[3]	reporting bias[4]	23/30 (76.7%)	0/0 (0%)	RR 0 (0 to 0)	0 fewer per 1000 (from 0 fewer to 0 fewer)	VERY LOW	CRITICAL
15 例的 CCS 积分 (follow – up mean 2 weeks; Better indicated by lower values)												
1	observational studies[1]	serious[1]	no serious inconsistency	serious[2]	serious[3]	reporting bias[4]	15	0	–	MD 0 higher (0 to 0 higher)	VERY LOW	NOT IMPORTANT
15 例的 CCS 有效率 (follow – up mean 2 weeks)												
1	observational studies[1]	serious[1]	no serious inconsistency	serious[2]	serious[3]	reporting bias[4]	14/15 (93.3%)	0/0 (0%)	RR 0 (0 to 0)	0 fewer per 1000 (from 0 fewer to 0 fewer)	VERY LOW	CRITICAL

续表

No of studies	Quality assessment						No of patients		Summary of findings			Importance
	Design	Limitations	Inconsistency	Indirectness	Imprecision	Other considerations	深刺天枢	control	Effect		Quality	
									Relative (95% CI)	Absolute		
15 例的 CTT 结果（follow-up mean 2 weeks; Better indicated by lower values）												
1	observational studies[1]	serious[1]	no serious inconsistency	serious[2]	serious[3]	reporting bias[4]	15	0	-	mean 0 higher（0 to 0 higher）	VERY LOW	IMPORTANT
15 例的 CCT 有效率（follow-up mean 2 weeks）												
1	observational studies[1]	serious[1]	no serious inconsistency	serious[2]	serious[3]	reporting bias[4]	12/15 （80%）	0/0（0%）	RR 0（0 to 0）	0 fewer per 1000（from 0 fewer to 0 fewer）	VERY LOW	CRITICAL

1 Case Series.

2 主观性指标。

3 样本量较小。

4 只有一篇文献纳入。

Author (s):

Date: 2011 – 08 – 08

Question: 轮流电针两组穴 for 肠慢传输型便秘

Settings:

Bibliography:

No of studies	Quality assessment						No of patients		Summary of findings		Quality	Importance
	Design	Limitations	Inconsistency	Indirectness	Imprecision	Other considerations	轮流电针两组穴	control	Relative (95% CI)	Effect — Absolute		
QOL 身体不适差值（follow – up mean 20 days；Better indicated by lower values）												
1	observational studies[1]	serious[1]	no serious inconsistency	serious[2]	serious[3]	reporting bias[4]	30	0	-	MD 0 higher (0 to 0 higher)	VERY LOW	IMPORTANT
QOL 心理不适（follow – up mean 20 days；Better indicated by lower values）												
1	observational studies[1]	serious[1]	no serious inconsistency	serious[2]	serious[3]	reporting bias[4]	30	0	-	mean 0 higher (0 to 0 higher)	VERY LOW	IMPORTANT
QOL 便秘相关的焦虑（follow – up mean 20 days）												
1	observational studies[1]	serious[1]	no serious inconsistency	serious[2]	serious[3]	reporting bias[4]	0/0 (0%)	0/0 (0%) 0%	RR 0 (0 to 0)	0 fewer per 1000 (from 0 fewer to 0 fewer) 0 fewer per 1000 (from 0 fewer to 0 fewer)	VERY LOW	IMPORTANT
QOL 满意度（follow – up mean 20 days）												
1	observational studies[1]	serious[1]	no serious inconsistency	serious[2]	serious[3]	reporting bias[4]	0/0 (0%)	0/0 (0%) 0%	RR 0 (0 to 0)	0 fewer per 1000 (from 0 fewer to 0 fewer) 0 fewer per 1000 (from 0 fewer to 0 fewer)	VERY LOW	CRITICAL
治疗结束有效率（follow – up mean 20 days）												
1	observational studies[1]	serious[1]	no serious inconsistency	serious[2]	serious[3]	reporting bias[4]	22/30 (73.3%)	0/0 (0%)	RR 0 (0 to 0)	0 fewer per 1000 (from 0 fewer to 0 fewer)	VERY LOW	CRITICAL

续表

No of studies	Quality assessment						No of patients		Summary of findings			
	Design	Limitations	Inconsistency	Indirectness	Imprecision	Other considerations	轮流电针两组穴	control	Effect		Quality	Importance
									Relative (95% CI)	Absolute		
治疗结束 1 个月有效率（follow – up mean 1 months）												
1	observational studies[1]	serious[1]	no serious in-consistency	serious[2]	serious[3]	reporting bias[4]	17/30 (56.7%)	0/0 (0%)	RR 0 (0 to 0)	0 fewer per 1000（from 0 fewer to 0 fewer）	VERY LOW	CRITICAL
治疗结束 3 个月有效率（follow – up mean 3 months）												
1	observational studies[1]	serious[1]	no serious in-consistency	serious[2]	serious[3]	reporting bias[4]	15/30 (50%)	0/0 (0%)	RR 0 (0 to 0)	0 fewer per 1000（from 0 fewer to 0 fewer）	VERY LOW	CRITICAL

1 Case Series.
2 主观性指标。
3 样本量小。
4 只纳入一篇文献。

Author（s）：

Date：2011 – 08 – 08

Question：润肠汤 + 埋线 VS 西沙必利片 for 慢传输型便秘

Settings：

Bibliography：

症状积分比较（follow – up mean 1 months；Better indicated by lower values）

No of studies	Quality assessment						No of patients		Summary of findings		Quality	Importance
	Design	Limitations	Inconsistency	Indirectness	Imprecision	Other considerations	润肠汤 + 埋线利片	润肠汤 + 埋线 VS 西沙必	Relative (95% CI)	Effect Absolute		
1	observational studies	serious[1]	no serious inconsistency	serious[2]	no serious imprecision	reporting bias[3]	49	48	–	SMD 1.23 higher (0.79 to 1.66 higher)	VERY LOW	NOT IMPORTANT

1 非随机同期对照。

2 主观指标。

3 只有一篇文献纳入。

Author（s）：

Date：2011 – 08 – 10

Question：针灸＋生物反馈 VS 盆底肌训练 for 盆底松弛综合征型便秘

Settings：

Bibliography：

No of studies	Quality assessment						No of patients		Summary of findings			Quality	Importance
	Design	Limitations	Inconsistency	Indirectness	Imprecision	Other considerations	针灸＋生物反馈 VS 盆底肌训练		Effect				
									Relative (95% CI)	Absolute			

有效率（follow – up mean 20 days）

No of studies	Design	Limitations	Inconsistency	Indirectness	Imprecision	Other considerations	针灸＋生物反馈 肌训练	VS 盆底	Relative (95% CI)	Absolute	Quality	Importance
1	observational studies	serious[1]	no serious inconsistency	serious[2]	serious[3]	reporting bias[4]	17/20 (85%)	4/20 (20%)	RR 4.25 (1.74 to 10.41)	650 more per 1000 (from 148 more to 1882 more)	VERY LOW	CRITICAL
								20%		650 more per 1000 (from 148 more to 1882 more)		

PAC – QOL 评分（follow – up mean 20 days；Better indicated by lower values）

No of studies	Design	Limitations	Inconsistency	Indirectness	Imprecision	Other considerations	针灸＋生物反馈 肌训练	VS 盆底	Relative (95% CI)	Absolute	Quality	Importance
1	observational studies	serious[1]	no serious inconsistency	serious[2]	serious[3]	reporting bias[4]	20	20	–	SMD 0.7 higher (0.06 to 1.34 higher)	VERY LOW	IMPORTANT

1 假 RCT。

2 主观性指标。

3 样本量小。

4 只纳入一篇文献。

Author（s）：

Date：2012 – 05 – 22

Question：穴位埋线 VS 手针 for 慢性便秘

Settings：

Bibliography：

No of studies	Quality assessment						No of patients		Summary of findings			
	Design	Limitations	Inconsistency	Indirectness	Imprecision	Other considerations	穴位埋线 VS 手针		Effect		Quality	Importance
									Relative (95% CI)	Absolute		
总有效率（follow – up mean 8 weeks；revman）												
1	randomised trials	serious[1]	no serious inconsistency	serious[2]	no serious imprecision	reporting bias[3]	68/72 (94.4%)	58/72 (80.6%)	RR 1.17 (1.03 to 1.33)	137 more per 1000 (from 24 more to 266 more)	VERY LOW	CRITICAL

1 分配隐藏及盲法存在缺陷。

2 主观性指标。

3 只纳入一个研究。

5.2 结果总结表（the summary of findings table，SoFs table）

手针 + 穴位注射 VS 药物 for 慢性便秘

Patient or population：patients with 慢性便秘
Settings：
Intervention：手针 + 穴位注射 VS 药物

Outcomes	Illustrative comparative risks* (95% CI)		Relative effect (95% CI)	No of Participants (studies)	Quality of the evidence (GRADE)	Comments
	Assumed risk	Corresponding risk				
	Control	手针 + 穴位注射 VS 药物				
	Study population					
总有效率 revman Follow – up: mean 4 weeks	682 per 1000	955 per 1000 (709 to 1000)	RR 1.4 (1.04 to 1.89)	45 (1 study)	⊕⊖⊖⊖ very low[1,2,3]	
	Medium risk population					
	682 per 1000	955 per 1000 (709 to 1000)				

* The basis for the assumed risk (e. g. the median control group risk across studies) is provided in footnotes. The corresponding risk (and its 95% confidence interval) is based on the assumed risk in the comparison group and the relative effect of the intervention (and its 95% CI).
CI: Confidence interval; RR: Risk ratio;

GRADE Working Group grades of evidence
High quality: Further research is very unlikely to change our confidence in the estimate of effect.
Moderate quality: Further research is likely to have an important impact on our confidence in the estimate of effect and may change the estimate.
Low quality: Further research is very likely to have an important impact on our confidence in the estimate of effect and is likely to change the estimate.
Very low quality: We are very uncertain about the estimate.

1 随机分组人员参与纳入病人；利益相关；未实施育法。
2 结局指标为主观性间接证据。
3 只有一篇文献。

指针＋穴位埋线 VS 药物 for 慢性便秘

Patient or population: patients with 慢性便秘
Settings:
Intervention: 指针＋穴位埋线 VS 药物

Outcomes	Illustrative comparative risks* (95% CI)		Relative effect (95% CI)	No of Participants (studies)	Quality of the evidence (GRADE)	Comments
	Assumed risk Control	Corresponding risk 指针＋穴位埋线 VS 药物				
总有效率 revman Follow－up: mean 5 weeks	Study population		RR 1.32 (1.02 to 1.69)	68 (1 study)	⊕⊖⊖⊖ very low[1,2,3]	
	700 per 1000	924 per 1000 (714 to 1000)				
	Medium risk population					
	700 per 1000	924 per 1000 (714 to 1000)				

* The basis for the assumed risk (e. g. the median control group risk across studies) is provided in footnotes. The corresponding risk (and its 95% confidence interval) is based on the assumed risk in the comparison group and the relative effect of the intervention (and its 95% CI).
CI: Confidence interval; RR: Risk ratio;

GRADE Working Group grades of evidence
High quality: Further research is very unlikely to change our confidence in the estimate of effect.
Moderate quality: Further research is likely to have an important impact on our confidence in the estimate of effect and may change the estimate.
Low quality: Further research is very likely to have an important impact on our confidence in the estimate of effect and is likely to change the estimate.
Very low quality: We are very uncertain about the estimate.

1 盲法天生设计缺陷，未分析试验本身存在的偏移可能性。
2 主观指标。
3 只有一个试验。

指针 + 穴位埋线 VS 药物 for 慢性便秘

Patient or population: patients with 慢性便秘
Settings:
Intervention: 指针 + 穴位埋线 VS 药物

Outcomes	Illustrative comparative risks* (95% CI)		Relative effect (95% CI)	No of Participants (studies)	Quality of the evidence (GRADE)	Comments
	Assumed risk Control	Corresponding risk 指针 + 穴位埋线 VS 药物				
	Study population					
总有效率 revman Follow – up: mean 5 weeks	700 per 1000	924 per 1000 (714 to 1000)	RR 1.32 (1.02 to 1.69)	68 (1 study)	⊕⊝⊝⊝ very low[1,2,3]	
	Medium risk population					
	700 per 1000	924 per 1000 (714 to 1000)				

* The basis for the assumed risk (e. g. the median control group risk across studies) is provided in footnotes. The corresponding risk (and its 95% confidence interval) is based on the assumed risk in the comparison group and the relative effect of the intervention (and its 95% CI).
CI: Confidence interval; RR: Risk ratio;

GRADE Working Group grades of evidence
High quality: Further research is very unlikely to change our confidence in the estimate of effect.
Moderate quality: Further research is likely to have an important impact on our confidence in the estimate of effect and may change the estimate.
Low quality: Further research is very likely to have an important impact on our confidence in the estimate of effect and is likely to change the estimate.
Very low quality: We are very uncertain about the estimate.

1 盲法天生设计缺陷，未分析试验本身存在的偏移可能性。
2 主观指标。
3 只有一个试验。

温针 + 中药汤剂 VS 药物 for 慢性便秘

Patient or population: patients with 慢性便秘
Settings:
Intervention: 温针 + 中药汤剂 VS 药物

Outcomes	Illustrative comparative risks* (95% CI)		Relative effect (95% CI)	No of Participants (studies)	Quality of the evidence (GRADE)	Comments
	Assumed risk	Corresponding risk				
	Control	温针 + 中药汤剂 VS 药物				
	Study population					
总有效率 revman Follow – up: mean 10 days	733 per 1000	968 per 1000 (770 to 1000)	RR 1.32 (1.05 to 1.65)	60 (1 study)	⊕⊝⊝⊝ very low[1,2,3]	
	Medium risk population					
	733 per 1000	968 per 1000 (770 to 1000)				

* The basis for the assumed risk (e. g. the median control group risk across studies) is provided in footnotes. The corresponding risk (and its 95% confidence interval) is based on the assumed risk in the comparison group and the relative effect of the intervention (and its 95% CI).
CI: Confidence interval; RR: Risk ratio;

GRADE Working Group grades of evidence
High quality: Further research is very unlikely to change our confidence in the estimate of effect.
Moderate quality: Further research is likely to have an important impact on our confidence in the estimate of effect and may change the estimate.
Low quality: Further research is very likely to have an important impact on our confidence in the estimate of effect and is likely to change the estimate.
Very low quality: We are very uncertain about the estimate.

1 盲法缺陷；分配隐藏缺陷。
2 结局指标以主观为主。
3 只有一篇文献。

耳穴压豆 VS 药物 for 慢性便秘

Patient or population: patients with 慢性便秘
Settings:
Intervention: 耳穴压豆 VS 药物

Outcomes	Illustrative comparative risks* (95% CI)		Relative effect (95% CI)	No of Participants (studies)	Quality of the evidence (GRADE)	Comments
	Assumed risk	Corresponding risk				
	Control	耳穴压豆 VS 药物				
有效率 revman Follow–up: mean 8 weeks	Study population		RR 1.08 (0.88 to 1.32)	60 (1 study)	⊕⊕⊝⊝ very low[1,2,3]	
	833 per 1000	900 per 1000 (733 to 1000)				
	Medium risk population					
	833 per 1000	900 per 1000 (733 to 1000)				
首次排便时间 Follow–up: mean 8 weeks		The mean 首次排便时间 in the intervention groups was 0.79 standard deviations lower (1.31 to 0.26 lower)		60 (1 study)	⊕⊕⊝⊝ low[1,3]	SMD −0.79 (−1.31 to −0.26)
治疗前后总积分差 Follow–up: mean 8 weeks		The mean 治疗前后总积分差 in the intervention groups was 0.71 standard deviations higher (0.19 to 1.24 higher)		60 (1 study)	⊕⊕⊝⊝ low[1,3]	SMD 0.71 (0.19 to 1.24)
治疗前后排便时间差 Follow–up: mean 8 weeks		The mean 治疗前后排便时间差 in the intervention groups was 0.3 standard deviations higher (0.21 lower to 0.81 higher)		60 (1 study)	⊕⊕⊝⊝ low[1,3]	SMD 0.3 (−0.21 to 0.81)
治疗前后排便速度差值 Follow–up: mean 8 weeks		The mean 治疗前后排便速度差值 in the intervention groups was 1.06 standard deviations higher (0.52 to 1.6 higher)		60 (1 study)	⊕⊕⊝⊝ low[1,3]	SMD 1.06 (0.52 to 1.6)
治疗前后大便性状差 Follow–up: mean 8 weeks		The mean 治疗前后大便性状差 in the intervention groups was 0.63 standard deviations higher (0.11 to 1.15 higher)		60 (1 study)	⊕⊕⊝⊝ low[1,2,3]	SMD 0.63 (0.11 to 1.15)
治疗前后排便难度积分差 Follow–up: mean 8 weeks		The mean 治疗前后排便难度积分差 in the intervention groups was 0.11 standard deviations higher (0.39 lower to 0.62 higher)		60 (1 study)	⊕⊕⊝⊝ low[1,2,3]	SMD 0.11 (−0.39 to 0.62)

续表

Outcomes	Illustrative comparative risks * (95% CI)		Relative effect (95% CI)	No of Participants (studies)	Quality of the evidence (GRADE)	Comments
	Assumed risk	Corresponding risk				
	Control	耳穴压豆 VS 药物				
治疗前后便意积分差 Follow－up: mean 8 weeks		The mean 治疗前后便意积分差 in the intervention groups was 0.45 standard deviations higher (0.06 lower to 0.97 higher)		60 (1 study)	⊕⊕⊖⊖ low[1,2,3]	SMD 0.45 (－0.06 to 0.97)

* The basis for the assumed risk (e. g. the median control group risk across studies) is provided in footnotes. The corresponding risk (and its 95% confidence interval) is based on the assumed risk in the comparison group and the relative effect of the intervention (and its 95% CI).
CI: Confidence interval; RR: Risk ratio;

GRADE Working Group grades of evidence
High quality: Further research is very unlikely to change our confidence in the estimate of effect.
Moderate quality: Further research is likely to have an important impact on our confidence in the estimate of effect and may change the estimate.
Low quality: Further research is very likely to have an important impact on our confidence in the estimate of effect and is likely to change the estimate.
Very low quality: We are very uncertain about the estimate.

1 分配隐藏、盲法缺陷。
2 结局以主观为主。
3 只有一个试验。

手针 VS 手针 for 慢性便秘

Patient or population: patients with 慢性便秘
Settings:
Intervention: 手针 VS 手针

Outcomes	Illustrative comparative risks * (95% CI)		Relative effect (95% CI)	No of Participants (studies)	Quality of the evidence (GRADE)	Comments
	Assumed risk	Corresponding risk				
	Control	手针 VS 手针				
有效率 revman Follow – up: mean 3 weeks	Study population		RR 1.09 (0.88 to 1.37)	62 (1 study)	⊕⊕⊝⊝ very low[1,2,3,4]	
	800 per 1000	872 per 1000 (704 to 1000)				
	Medium risk population					
	800 per 1000	872 per 1000 (704 to 1000)				
粪便性状正常率 revman Follow – up: mean 3 weeks	Study population		RR 1.17 (0.66 to 2.08)	62 (1 study)	⊕⊕⊝⊝ very low[2,3,4]	
	400 per 1000	468 per 1000 (264 to 832)				
	Medium risk population					
	400 per 1000	468 per 1000 (264 to 832)				
治疗前后症状总积分差 Follow – up: mean 3 weeks		The mean 治疗前后症状总积分差 in the intervention groups was 0.43 standard deviations higher (0.08 lower to 0.93 higher)		62 (1 study)	⊕⊕⊝⊝ low[1,2,3,4]	SMD 0.43 (−0.08 to 0.93)
治疗前后排便间隔时间差 Follow – up: mean 3 weeks		The mean 治疗前后排便间隔时间差 in the intervention groups was 0 standard deviations higher (0.5 lower to 0.5 higher)		62 (1 study)	⊕⊕⊕⊝ 	SMD 0 (−0.5 to 0.5)
治疗前后排便速度差 Follow – up: mean 3 weeks		The mean 治疗前后排便速度差 in the intervention groups was 1.53 standard deviations higher (0.96 to 2.1 higher)		62 (1 study)	⊕⊕⊝⊝ low[1,3,4]	SMD 1.53 (0.96 to 2.1)

Outcomes	Illustrative comparative risks* (95% CI) 手针 VS 手针		Relative effect (95% CI)	No of Participants (studies)	Quality of the evidence (GRADE)	Comments
	Assumed risk Control	Corresponding risk				
治疗前后排便难度差 Follow – up: mean 3 weeks		The mean 治疗前后排便难度差 in the intervention groups was 0.31 standard deviations lower (0.81 lower to 0.19 higher)		62 (1 study)	⊕⊕⊖⊖ low[1,2,3,4]	SMD –0.31 (–0.81 to 0.19)
治疗前后排便性状差值 Follow – up: mean 3 weeks		The mean 治疗前后排便性状差值 in the intervention groups was 0.62 standard deviations higher (0.11 to 1.13 higher)		62 (1 study)	⊕⊕⊖⊖ low[1,2,3,4]	SMD 0.62 (0.11 to 1.13)
治疗前后便意差值 Follow – up: mean 3 weeks		The mean 治疗前后便意差值 in the intervention groups was 0 standard deviations higher (0.5 lower to 0.5 higher)		62 (1 study)	⊕⊕⊖⊖ low[1,2,3,4]	SMD 0 (–0.5 to 0.5)
治疗前后焦虑自评量 SAS 表差值 Follow – up: mean 3 weeks		The mean 治疗前后焦虑自评量 SAS 表差值 in the intervention groups was 1.61 standard deviations higher (1.03 to 2.18 higher)		62 (1 study)	⊕⊕⊖⊖ low[1,2,3,4]	SMD 1.61 (1.03 to 2.18)

* The basis for the assumed risk (e. g. the median control group risk across studies) is provided in footnotes. The corresponding risk (and its 95% confidence interval) is based on the assumed risk in the comparison group and the relative effect of the intervention (and its 95% CI) .
CI: Confidence interval; RR: Risk ratio;

GRADE Working Group grades of evidence
High quality: Further research is very unlikely to change our confidence in the estimate of effect.
Moderate quality: Further research is likely to have an important impact on our confidence in the estimate of effect and may change the estimate.
Low quality: Further research is very likely to have an important impact on our confidence in the estimate of effect and is likely to change the estimate.
Very low quality: We are very uncertain about the estimate.

1 分配隐藏、盲法缺陷。
2 主观指标。
3 样本量小，可信区间宽。
4 只有一个试验纳入。

灸法 VS 药物 for 慢性便秘

Patient or population: patients with 慢性便秘
Settings:
Intervention: 灸法 VS 药物

Outcomes	Illustrative comparative risks* (95% CI)		Relative effect (95% CI)	No of Participants (studies)	Quality of the evidence (GRADE)	Comments
	Assumed risk	Corresponding risk				
	Control	灸法 VS 药物				
	Study population					
总有效率 revman Follow – up: mean 2 months	533 per 1000	863 per 1000 (602 to 1000)	RR 1.62 (1.13 to 2.34)	60 (1 study)	⊕⊖⊖⊖ very low[1,2,3,4]	
	Medium risk population					
	533 per 1000	863 per 1000 (602 to 1000)				

* The basis for the assumed risk (e. g. the median control group risk across studies) is provided in footnotes. The corresponding risk (and its 95% confidence interval) is based on the assumed risk in the comparison group and the relative effect of the intervention (and its 95% CI).
CI: Confidence interval; RR: Risk ratio;

GRADE Working Group grades of evidence
High quality: Further research is very unlikely to change our confidence in the estimate of effect.
Moderate quality: Further research is likely to have an important impact on our confidence in the estimate of effect and may change the estimate.
Low quality: Further research is very likely to have an important impact on our confidence in the estimate of effect and is likely to change the estimate.
Very low quality: We are very uncertain about the estimate.

1 盲法，分配隐藏缺陷。
2 主观指标。
3 样本量小，可信区间宽。
4 只有一个试验被纳入。

电针＋灸法 VS 电针 for 慢性便秘

Patient or population: patients with 慢性便秘
Settings:
Intervention: 电针＋灸法 VS 电针

Outcomes	Illustrative comparative risks* (95% CI)		Relative effect (95% CI)	No of Participants (studies)	Quality of the evidence (GRADE)	Comments
	Assumed risk	Corresponding risk				
	Control	电针＋灸法 VS 电针				
	Study population					
有效率 revman Follow－up: mean 20 days	520 per 1000	702 per 1000 (510 to 967)	RR 1.35 (0.98 to 1.86)	100 (1 study)	⊕⊕⊝⊝ low[1,2]	
	Medium risk population					
	520 per 1000	702 per 1000 (510 to 967)				
治疗前后生活质量 PAC－QOL 差值 Follow－up: mean 20 days		The mean 治疗前后生活质量 PAC－QOL 差值 in the intervention groups was 0.53 standard deviations higher (0.13 to 0.93 higher)		100 (1 study)	⊕⊕⊝⊝ low[1,2,3]	SMD 0.53 (0.13 to 0.93)
治疗前后心理症状评分 SCL－90 差值 Follow－up: mean 20 days		The mean 治疗前后心理症状评分 SCL－90 差值 in the intervention groups was 0.19 standard deviations higher (0.21 lower to 0.58 higher)		100 (1 study)	⊕⊕⊝⊝ low[1,2,3]	SMD 0.19 (－0.21 to 0.58)

*The basis for the assumed risk (e.g. the median control group risk across studies) is provided in footnotes. The corresponding risk (and its 95% confidence interval) is based on the assumed risk in the comparison group and the relative effect of the intervention (and its 95% CI).
CI: Confidence interval; RR: Risk ratio;

GRADE Working Group grades of evidence
High quality: Further research is very unlikely to change our confidence in the estimate of effect.
Moderate quality: Further research is likely to have an important impact on our confidence in the estimate of effect and may change the estimate.
Low quality: Further research is very likely to have an important impact on our confidence in the estimate of effect and is likely to change the estimate.
Very low quality: We are very uncertain about the estimate.

1 样本量小，95%CI 宽。
2 只有一个试验。
3 主观性指标。

电针 VS sham needle for 慢性便秘

Patient or population: patients with 慢性便秘
Settings:
Intervention: 电针 VS sham needle

Outcomes	Illustrative comparative risks* (95% CI)		Relative effect (95% CI)	No of Participants (studies)	Quality of the evidence (GRADE)	Comments
	Assumed risk	Corresponding risk				
	Control	电针 VS sham needle				
有效率 revman Follow – up: mean 4 weeks	Study population		RR 1.54 (1.34 to 1.78)	255 (1 study)	⊕⊕⊝⊝ low[1,2]	
	612 per 1000	942 per 1000 (820 to 1000)				
	Medium risk population					
	612 per 1000	942 per 1000 (820 to 1000)				
治疗 1 周症状积分差值 Follow – up: mean 4 weeks		The mean 治疗 1 周症状积分差值 in the intervention groups was 8.25 standard deviations higher (7.48 to 9.01 higher)		255 (1 study)	⊕⊕⊝⊝ low[1,2]	SMD 8.25 (7.48 to 9.01)
治疗 2 周症状积分差值 Follow – up: mean 4 weeks		The mean 治疗 2 周症状积分差值 in the intervention groups was 11.47 standard deviations higher (10.44 to 12.5 higher)		255 (1 study)	⊕⊕⊝⊝ low[1,2]	SMD 11.47 (10.44 to 12.5)
治疗 3 周症状积分差值 Follow – up: mean 4 weeks		The mean 治疗 3 周症状积分差值 in the intervention groups was 17.27 standard deviations higher (15.74 to 18.8 higher)		255 (1 study)	⊕⊕⊝⊝ low[1,2]	SMD 17.27 (15.74 to 18.8)
治疗 4 周症状积分差值 Follow – up: mean 4 weeks		The mean 治疗 4 周症状积分差值 in the intervention groups was 24.81 standard deviations higher (22.63 to 27 higher)		255 (1 study)	⊕⊕⊝⊝ low[1,2]	SMD 24.81 (22.63 to 27)
治疗后 1 个月随访症状积分差值 Follow – up: mean 4 weeks		The mean 治疗后 1 个月随访症状积分差值 in the intervention groups was 12.4 standard deviations higher (11.29 to 13.52 higher)		255 (1 study)	⊕⊕⊝⊝ low[1,2]	SMD 12.4 (11.29 to 13.52)

续表

Outcomes	Illustrative comparative risks * (95% CI)		Relative effect (95% CI)	No of Participants (studies)	Quality of the evidence (GRADE)	Comments
	Assumed risk Control	Corresponding risk 电针 VS sham needle				
治疗后 3 个月随访症状积分差值 Follow – up: mean 4 weeks		The mean 治疗后 3 个月随访症状积分差值 in the intervention groups was 11.73 standard deviations higher (10.68 to 12.79 higher)		255 (1 study)	⊕⊕⊖⊖ low[1,2]	SMD 11.73 (10.68 to 12.79)
治疗前后 72 小时结肠标志物排除率差值 Follow – up: mean 4 weeks		The mean 治疗前后 72 小时结肠标志物排除率差值 in the intervention groups was 1.73 standard deviations higher (1.44 to 2.02 higher)		255 (1 study)	⊕⊕⊕⊖ moderate[2]	SMD 1.73 (1.44 to 2.02)

* The basis for the assumed risk (e. g. the median control group risk across studies) is provided in footnotes. The corresponding risk (and its 95% confidence interval) is based on the assumed risk in the comparison group and the relative effect of the intervention (and its 95% CI).

CI: Confidence interval; RR: Risk ratio;

GRADE Working Group grades of evidence

High quality: Further research is very unlikely to change our confidence in the estimate of effect.

Moderate quality: Further research is likely to have an important impact on our confidence in the estimate of effect and may change the estimate.

Low quality: Further research is very likely to have an important impact on our confidence in the estimate of effect and is likely to change the estimate.

Very low quality: We are very uncertain about the estimate.

1 主观性指标。

2 只有一个试验纳入。

针刺 + 灸法 VS 生物反馈 for 慢性便秘

Patient or population: patients with 慢性便秘
Settings:
Intervention: 针刺 + 灸法 VS 生物反馈

Outcomes	Illustrative comparative risks* (95% CI)		Relative effect (95% CI)	No of Participants (studies)	Quality of the evidence (GRADE)	Comments
	Assumed risk	Corresponding risk				
	Control	针刺 + 灸法 VS 生物反馈				
有效率 revman Follow – up: mean 2 weeks	Study population		RR 1.67 (0.75 to 3.71)	40 (1 study)	⊕⊖⊖⊖ very low[1,2,3]	
	300 per 1000	501 per 1000 (225 to 1000)				
	Medium risk population					
	300 per 1000	501 per 1000 (225 to1000)				
治疗前后 PAC – QOL 评分差值 Follow – up: mean 2 weeks	The mean 治疗前后 PAC – QOL 评分差值 in the intervention groups was 0.16 standard deviations higher (0.46 lower to 0.78 higher)			40 (1 study)	⊕⊖⊖⊖ very low[1,2,3,4]	SMD 0.16 (– 0.46 to 0.78)

* The basis for the assumed risk (e. g. the median control group risk across studies) is provided in footnotes. The corresponding risk (and its 95% confidence interval) is based on the assumed risk in the comparison group and the relative effect of the intervention (and its 95% CI).
CI: Confidence interval; RR: Risk ratio;

GRADE Working Group grades of evidence
High quality: Further research is very unlikely to change our confidence in the estimate of effect.
Moderate quality: Further research is likely to have an important impact on our confidence in the estimate of effect and may change the estimate.
Low quality: Further research is very likely to have an important impact on our confidence in the estimate of effect and is likely to change the estimate.
Very low quality: We are very uncertain about the estimate.

1 主观指标。
2 样本量小。
3 只有一篇文献纳入。
4 分配隐藏、盲法缺陷。

针刺 + 灸法 + 生物反馈 VS 生物反馈 for 慢性便秘

Patient or population: patients with 慢性便秘
Settings:
Intervention: 针刺 + 灸法 + 生物反馈 VS 生物反馈

Outcomes	Illustrative comparative risks * (95% CI)		Relative effect (95% CI)	No of Participants (studies)	Quality of the evidence (GRADE)	Comments
	Assumed risk Control	Corresponding risk 针刺 + 灸法 + 生物反馈 VS 生物反馈				
	Study population					
有效率 revman Follow－up: mean 2 weeks	300 per 1000	651 per 1000 (309 to 1000)	RR 2.17 (1.03 to 4.55)	40 (1 study)	⊕⊝⊝⊝ very low[1,2,3,4]	
	Medium risk population					
	300 per 1000	651 per 1000 (309 to 1000)				
治疗前后 PAC－QOL 评分差值 Follow－up: mean 2 weeks		The mean 治疗前后 PAC－QOL 评分差值 in the intervention groups was 0.4 standard deviations higher (0.22 lower to 1.03 higher) .		40 (1 study)	⊕⊝⊝⊝ very low[1,2,3,4]	SMD 0.4 (－0.22 to 1.03)

* The basis for the assumed risk (e. g. the median control group risk across studies) is provided in footnotes. The corresponding risk (and its 95% confidence interval) is based on the assumed risk in the comparison group and the relative effect of the intervention (and its 95% CI) .
CI: Confidence interval; RR: Risk ratio;

GRADE Working Group grades of evidence
High quality: Further research is very unlikely to change our confidence in the estimate of effect.
Moderate quality: Further research is likely to have an important impact on our confidence in the estimate of effect and may change the estimate.
Low quality: Further research is very likely to have an important impact on our confidence in the estimate of effect and is likely to change the estimate.
Very low quality: We are very uncertain about the estimate.

1 分配隐藏、盲法缺陷。
2 主观指标。
3 样本量小。
4 只有一篇文献纳入。

91

针刺 + 灸法 + 生物反馈 VS 针刺 + 灸法 for 慢性便秘

Patient or population: patients with 慢性便秘
Settings:
Intervention: 针刺 + 灸法 + 生物反馈 VS 针刺 + 灸法

Outcomes	Illustrative comparative risks * (95% CI)		Relative effect (95% CI)	No of Participants (studies)	Quality of the evidence (GRADE)	Comments
	Assumed risk	Corresponding risk				
	Control	针刺 + 灸法 + 生物反馈 VS 针刺 + 灸法				
	Study population					
有效率 revman Follow – up: mean 2 weeks	500 per 1000	650 per 1000 (375 to 1000)	RR 1.3 (0.75 to 2.24)	40 (1 study)	⊕⊖⊖⊖ very low[1,2,3,4]	
	Medium risk population					
	500 per 1000	650 per 1000 (375 to 1000)				
治疗前后 PAC – QOL 评分差值 Follow – up: mean 2 weeks	The mean 治疗前后 PAC – QOL 评分差值 in the intervention groups was 0.28 standard deviations higher (0.34 lower to 0.9 higher)			40 (1 study)	⊕⊖⊖⊖ very low[1,2,3,4]	SMD 0.28 (– 0.34 to 0.9)

* The basis for the assumed risk (e. g. the median control group risk across studies) is provided in footnotes. The corresponding risk (and its 95% confidence interval) is based on the assumed risk in the comparison group and the relative effect of the intervention (and its 95% CI).
CI: Confidence interval; RR: Risk ratio;

GRADE Working Group grades of evidence
High quality: Further research is very unlikely to change our confidence in the estimate of effect.
Moderate quality: Further research is likely to have an important impact on our confidence in the estimate of effect and may change the estimate.
Low quality: Further research is very likely to have an important impact on our confidence in the estimate of effect and is likely to change the estimate.
Very low quality: We are very uncertain about the estimate.

1 盲法，分配隐藏缺陷。
2 主观指标。
3 样本量小。
4 只纳入一篇文献。

穴位埋线 VS 药物 for 慢性便秘

Patient or population: patients with 慢性便秘
Settings:
Intervention: 穴位埋线 VS 药物

Outcomes	Illustrative comparative risks* (95% CI) 穴位埋线 VS 药物		Relative effect (95% CI)	No of Participants (studies)	Quality of the evidence (GRADE)	Comments
	Assumed risk Control	Corresponding risk				
治疗 2 周后有效率 revman Follow – up: mean 2 weeks	Study population 733 per 1000 Medium risk population 733 per 1000	909 per 1000 (770 to 1000) 909 per 1000 (770 to 1000)	RR 1.24 (1.05 to 1.47)	120 (2 studies)	⊕⊕⊕⊝ low[1,2]	
治疗 2 周后有效率 – 脾俞 + 大肠俞埋线 VS 莫沙必利 revman Follow – up: mean 2 weeks	Study population 767 per 1000 Medium risk population 767 per 1000	897 per 1000 (713 to 1000) 897 per 1000 (713 to 1000)	RR 1.17 (0.93 to 1.48)	60 (1 study)	⊕⊝⊝⊝ very low[1,2,3,4]	
治疗 2 周后有效率 – 天元 + 大肠俞 + 关元 + 足三里 VS 莫沙必利 revman Follow – up: mean 2 weeks	Study population 700 per 1000 Medium risk population 700 per 1000	931 per 1000 (728 to 1000) 931 per 1000 (728 to 1000)	RR 1.33 (1.04 to 1.72)	60 (1 study)	⊕⊝⊝⊝ very low[1,2,4]	
治疗 4 周后有效率 revman Follow – up: mean 4 weeks	Study population 533 per 1000 Medium risk population 533 per 1000	863 per 1000 (602 to 1000) 863 per 1000 (602 to 1000)	RR 1.62 (1.13 to 2.34)	60 (1 study)	⊕⊝⊝⊝ very low[2,3,4]	

续表

Outcomes	Illustrative comparative risks* (95% CI)		Relative effect (95% CI)	No of Participants (studies)	Quality of the evidence (GRADE)	Comments
	Assumed risk Control	Corresponding risk 穴位埋线 VS 药物				
治疗结束后30天有效率 revman Follow – up: mean 30 days	Study population 11 per 1000 Medium risk population 11 per 1000	975 per 1000 (139 to 1000) 975 per 1000 (139 to 1000)	RR 88.6 (12.6 to 622.85)	181 (1 study)	⊕⊝⊝⊝ very low[1,2,4]	
治疗1次结束后3个月有效率 revman Follow – up: mean 3 months	Study population 11 per 1000 Medium risk population 11 per 1000	975 per 1000 (139 to 1000) 975 per 1000 (139 to 1000)	RR 88.6 (12.6 to 622.85)	181 (1 study)	⊕⊝⊝⊝ very low[1,2,4]	
排便间隔时间改善率 revman Follow – up: mean 4 weeks	Study population 897 per 1000 Medium risk population 897 per 1000	897 per 1000 (745 to 1000) 897 per 1000 (745 to 1000)	RR 1 (0.83 to 1.19)	57 (1 study)	⊕⊕⊝⊝ low[3,4]	
排便时间改善率 revman Follow – up: mean 4 weeks	Study population 583 per 1000 Medium risk population 583 per 1000	857 per 1000 (583 to 1000) 857 per 1000 (583 to 1000)	RR 1.47 (1 to 2.15)	45 (1 study)	⊕⊕⊝⊝ low[3,4]	
粪便性质改善率 revman Follow – up: mean 4 weeks	Study population 630 per 1000 Medium risk population 630 per 1000	788 per 1000 (554 to 1000) 788 per 1000 (554 to 1000)	RR 1.25 (0.88 to 1.77)	55 (1 study)	⊕⊝⊝⊝ very low[2,3,4]	

续表

Outcomes	Illustrative comparative risks* (95% CI)		Relative effect (95% CI)	No of Participants (studies)	Quality of the evidence (GRADE)	Comments
	Assumed risk Control	Corresponding risk 穴位埋线 VS 药物				
排便困难程度改善率 revman Follow – up: mean 4 weeks	Study population 300 per 1000 Medium risk population 300 per 1000	600 per 1000 (324 to 1000) 600 per 1000 (324 to 1000)	RR 2 (1.08 to 3.72)	60 (1 study)	⊕⊖⊖⊖ very low[2,3,4]	
兼症改善率 revman Follow – up: mean 4 weeks	Study population 552 per 1000 Medium risk population 552 per 1000	767 per 1000 (519 to 1000) 767 per 1000 (519 to 1000)	RR 1.39 (0.94 to 2.06)	55 (1 study)	⊕⊖⊖⊖ very low[2,3,4]	
治疗前后大便性状差值 Follow – up: mean 2 weeks		The mean 治疗前后大便性状差值 in the intervention groups was 1.31 standard deviations higher (0.75 to 1.87 higher)		60 (1 study)	⊕⊖⊖⊖ very low[1,2,4]	SMD 1.31 (0.75 to 1.87)
治疗前后每周排便次数值 Follow – up: mean 2 weeks		The mean 治疗前后每周排便次数值 in the intervention groups was 0.21 standard deviations lower (0.71 lower to 0.3 higher)		60 (1 study)	⊕⊕⊖⊖ low[1,4]	SMD – 0.21 (– 0.71 to 0.3)
治疗 4 次结束后 3 个月有效率 revman Follow – up: mean 3 months	811 per 1000	908 per 1000 (827 to 1000)	RR 1.12 (1.02 to 1.24)	264 (1 study)	⊕⊕⊖⊖ low[2,4]	
治疗结束后 6 个月有效率 revman Follow – up: mean 6 months	712 per 1000	897 per 1000 (790 to 1000)	RR 1.26 (1.11 to 1.42)	264 (1 study)	⊕⊕⊖⊖ low[2,4]	

* The basis for the assumed risk (e. g. the median control group risk across studies) is provided in footnotes. The corresponding risk (and its 95% confidence interval) is based on the assumed risk in the comparison group and the relative effect of the intervention (and its 95% CI) .

CI: Confidence interval; RR: Risk ratio;

GRADE Working Group grades of evidence

High quality: Further research is very unlikely to change our confidence in the estimate of effect.

Moderate quality: Further research is likely to have an important impact on our confidence in the estimate of effect and may change the estimate.

Low quality: Further research is very likely to have an important impact on our confidence in the estimate of effect and is likely to change the estimate.

Very low quality: We are very uncertain about the estimate.

1 分配隐藏及盲法缺陷。
2 主观性指标。
3 分配隐藏缺陷。
4 只纳入一篇文献。

手针 VS 药物 for 慢性便秘

Patient or population: patients with 慢性便秘
Settings:
Intervention: 手针 VS 药物

Outcomes	Illustrative comparative risks* (95% CI)		Relative effect (95% CI)	No of Participants (studies)	Quality of the evidence (GRADE)	Comments
	Assumed risk Control	Corresponding risk 手针 VS 药物				
开始治疗 1 个月后总有效率 revman	Study population		RR 1.07 (0.96 to 1.19)	207 (2 studies)	⊕⊕⊕⊝ very low[1,2,3]	
	892 per 1000	954 per 1000 (856 to 1000)				
	Medium risk population					
	887 per 1000	949 per 1000 (852 to 1000)				
开始治疗 1 个月后总有效率 – 手针背俞穴 VS 麻子仁丸 revman Follow – up: mean 3 weeks	Study population		RR 1.14 (1 to 1.3)	87 (1 study)	⊕⊕⊕⊝ low[3,4]	
	857 per 1000	977 per 1000 (857 to 1000)				
	Medium risk population					
	857 per 1000	977 per 1000 (857 to 1000)				
开始治疗 1 个月后总有效率 – 手针三其穴 VS 西沙必利 + 麻仁润肠丸 revman Follow – up: mean 15 days	Study population		RR 1.02 (0.92 to 1.13)	120 (1 study)	⊕⊕⊕⊝ very low[1,3,4]	
	917 per 1000	935 per 1000 (844 to 1000)				
	Medium risk population					
	917 per 1000	935 per 1000 (844 to 1000)				
开始治疗 1 个月后痊愈率 revman Follow – up: mean 3 weeks	Study population		RR 1.8 (1.14 to 2.86)	87 (1 study)	⊕⊕⊕⊝ low[3,5]	
	357 per 1000	643 per 1000 (407 to 1000)				
	Medium risk population					
	357 per 1000	643 per 1000 (407 to 1000)				

Outcomes	Illustrative comparative risks* (95% CI)		Relative effect (95% CI)	No of Participants (studies)	Quality of the evidence (GRADE)	Comments
	Assumed risk Control	Corresponding risk 手针 VS 药物				
开始治疗 4 个月后总有效率 revman Follow – up: mean 3 weeks	Study population		RR 1.67 (1.3 to 2.14)	87 (1 study)	⊕⊕⊕⊖ low[3,5]	
	595 per 1000	994 per 1000 (773 to 1000)				
	Medium risk population					
	595 per 1000	994 per 1000 (773 to 1000)				
开始治疗 4 个月后痊愈率 revman Follow – up: mean 3 weeks	Study population		RR 2.97 (1.75 to 5.05)	87 (1 study)	⊕⊕⊕⊖ low[3,5]	
	262 per 1000	778 per 1000 (459 to 1000)				
	Medium risk population					
	262 per 1000	778 per 1000 (459 to 1000)				
治疗 10 次便秘评分差值 Follow – up: mean 20 days	The mean 治疗 10 次便秘评分差值 in the intervention groups was 0.94 standard deviations higher (0.45 to 1.44 higher)			70 (1 study)	⊕⊕⊕⊖ low[3,5]	
治疗 20 次便秘评分差值 Follow – up: mean 20 days	The mean 治疗 20 次便秘评分差值 in the intervention groups was 3.68 standard deviations higher (2.42 to 4.94 higher)			70 (1 study)	⊕⊕⊕⊖ low[3,5]	

* The basis for the assumed risk (e. g. the median control group risk across studies) is provided in footnotes. The corresponding risk (and its 95% confidence interval) is based on the assumed risk in the comparison group and the relative effect of the intervention (and its 95% CI).
CI: Confidence interval; RR: Risk ratio;

GRADE Working Group grades of evidence
High quality: Further research is very unlikely to change our confidence in the estimate of effect.
Moderate quality: Further research is likely to have an important impact on our confidence in the estimate of effect and may change the estimate.
Low quality: Further research is very likely to have an important impact on our confidence in the estimate of effect and is likely to change the estimate.
Very low quality: We are very uncertain about the estimate.

1 盲法、分配隐藏缺陷。
2 去掉低质量、权重大文献后结果逆转。
3 主观指标。
4 只有一篇文献纳入亚组。
5 只有一篇文章纳入。

电针 VS 电针 for 慢性便秘

Patient or population: patients with 慢性便秘
Settings:
Intervention: 电针 VS 电针

Outcomes	Illustrative comparative risks* (95% CI)		Relative effect (95% CI)	No of Participants (studies)	Quality of the evidence (GRADE)	Comments
	Assumed risk Control	Corresponding risk 电针 VS 电针				
治疗 1 周后排便次数差值 Follow－up: mean 4 weeks		The mean 治疗 1 周后排便次数差值 in the intervention groups was 0.81 standard deviations higher (0.3 to 1.32 higher)		72 (1 study)	⊕⊕⊕⊝ moderate[1]	SMD 0.81 (0.3 to 1.32)
治疗 2 周后排便次数差值 Follow－up: mean 4 weeks		The mean 治疗 2 周后排便次数差值 in the intervention groups was 0.92 standard deviations higher (0.41 to 1.43 higher)		72 (1 study)	⊕⊕⊕⊝ moderate[1]	SMD 0.92 (0.41 to 1.43)
治疗 3 周后排便次数差值 Follow－up: mean 4 weeks		The mean 治疗 3 周后排便次数差值 in the intervention groups was 1.09 standard deviations higher (0.57 to 1.62 higher)		72 (1 study)	⊕⊕⊕⊝ moderate[1]	SMD 1.09 (0.57 to 1.62)
治疗 4 周后排便次数差值 Follow－up: mean 4 weeks		The mean 治疗 4 周后排便次数差值 in the intervention groups was 0.93 standard deviations higher (0.13 lower to 1.98 higher)		131 (2 studies)	⊕⊕⊕⊝ moderate[2]	SMD 0.93 (－0.13 to 1.98)
治疗结束后 4 周排便次数差值 Follow－up: mean 4 weeks		The mean 治疗结束后 4 周排便次数差值 in the intervention groups was 1.44 standard deviations higher (0.89 to 1.98 higher)		72 (1 study)	⊕⊕⊕⊝ moderate[1]	SMD 1.44 (0.89 to 1.98)
治疗结束后 12 周后排便次数差值 Follow－up: mean 4 weeks		The mean 治疗结束后 12 周后排便次数差值 in the intervention groups was 0.94 standard deviations higher (0.42 to 1.45 higher)		72 (1 study)	⊕⊕⊕⊝ moderate[1]	SMD 0.94 (0.42 to 1.45)
治疗结束后 6 个月后排便次数差值 Follow－up: mean 4 weeks		The mean 治疗结束后 6 个月后排便次数差值 in the intervention groups was 1.31 standard deviations higher (0.77 to 1.85 higher)		72 (1 study)	⊕⊕⊕⊝ moderate[1]	SMD 1.31 (0.77 to 1.85)

Outcomes	Illustrative comparative risks* (95% CI)		Relative effect (95% CI)	No of Participants (studies)	Quality of the evidence (GRADE)	Comments
	Assumed risk Control	Corresponding risk 电针 VS 电针				
治疗1周便秘评分差值 Follow-up: mean 4 weeks		The mean 治疗1周便秘评分值 in the intervention groups was 0.23 standard deviations higher (0.14 lower to 0.6 higher)		132 (2 studies)	⊕⊕⊕⊝ moderate[3]	SMD 0.23 (-0.14 to 0.6)
治疗1周便秘评分差值 - 深刺 天枢 VS 浅刺天枢 Follow-up: mean 4 weeks		The mean 治疗1周便秘评分值 - 深刺天枢 VS 浅刺天枢 in the intervention groups was 0.42 standard deviations higher (0.08 lower to 0.91 higher)		72 (1 study)	⊕⊕⊝⊝ low[1,3]	SMD 0.42 (-0.08 to 0.91)
治疗1周便秘评分差值 - 低频 电针 VS 高频电针 Follow-up: mean 4 weeks		The mean 治疗1周便秘评分值 - 低频电针 VS 高频电针 in the intervention groups was 0.04 standard deviations higher (0.47 lower to 0.54 higher)		60 (1 study)	⊕⊕⊝⊝ low[1,3]	SMD 0.04 (-0.47 to 0.54)
治疗2周便秘评分差值 Follow-up: mean 4 weeks		The mean 治疗2周便秘评分差值 in the intervention groups was 0.18 standard deviations higher (0.17 lower to 0.53 higher)		132 (2 studies)	⊕⊕⊕⊝ moderate[3]	SMD 0.18 (-0.17 to 0.53)
治疗2周便秘评分差值 - 深刺 天枢 VS 浅刺天枢 Follow-up: mean 4 weeks		The mean 治疗2周便秘评分值 - 深刺天枢 VS 浅刺天枢 in the intervention groups was 0.35 standard deviations higher (0.15 lower to 0.84 higher)		72 (1 study)	⊕⊕⊝⊝ low[1,3]	SMD 0.35 (-0.15 to 0.84)
治疗2周便秘评分差值 - 低频 电针 VS 高频电针 Follow-up: mean 4 weeks		The mean 治疗2周便秘评分值 - 低频电针 VS 高频电针 in the intervention groups was 0 standard deviations higher (0.51 lower to 0.51 higher)		60 (1 study)	⊕⊕⊝⊝ low[1,3]	SMD 0 (-0.51 to 0.51)
治疗3周便秘评分差值 Follow-up: mean 4 weeks		The mean 治疗3周便秘评分差值 in the intervention groups was 1.1 standard deviations higher (0.79 lower to 2.99 higher)		132 (2 studies)	⊕⊕⊕⊝ moderate[3]	SMD 1.1 (-0.79 to 2.99)
治疗3周便秘评分差值 - 深刺 天枢 VS 浅刺天枢 Follow-up: mean 4 weeks		The mean 治疗3周便秘评分值 - 深刺天枢 VS 浅刺天枢 in the intervention groups was 2.07 standard deviations higher (1.47 to 2.67 higher)		72 (1 study)	⊕⊕⊝⊝ low[1,3]	SMD 2.07 (1.47 to 2.67)
治疗3周便秘评分差值 - 低频 电针 VS 高频电针 Follow-up: mean 4 weeks		The mean 治疗3周便秘评分值 - 低频电针 VS 高频电针 in the intervention groups was 0.14 standard deviations higher (0.37 lower to 0.65 higher)		60 (1 study)	⊕⊕⊝⊝ low[1,3]	SMD 0.14 (-0.37 to 0.65)

续表

Outcomes	Illustrative comparative risks* (95% CI)		Relative effect (95% CI)	No of Participants (studies)	Quality of the evidence (GRADE)	Comments
	Assumed risk Control	Corresponding risk 电针 VS 电针				
治疗 4 周便秘评分差值 Follow－up: mean 4 weeks		The mean 治疗 4 周便秘评分差值 in the intervention groups was 0.57 standard deviations higher (0.21 to 0.92 higher)		261 (5 studies)	⊕⊕⊕⊖ moderate[3]	SMD 0.57 (0.21 to 0.92)
治疗 4 周便秘评分差值 － 深刺天枢 VS 浅刺天枢 Follow－up: mean 4 weeks		The mean 治疗 4 周便秘评分差值 － 深刺天枢 VS 浅刺天枢 in the intervention groups was 0.72 standard deviations higher (0.42 to 1.02 higher)		201 (4 studies)	⊕⊕⊖⊖ low[1,3]	SMD 0.72 (0.42 to 1.02)
治疗 4 周便秘评分差值 － 低频电针 VS 高频电针 Follow－up: mean 4 weeks		The mean 治疗 4 周便秘评分差值 － 低频电针 VS 高频电针 in the intervention groups was 0.08 standard deviations higher (0.43 lower to 0.59 higher)		60 (1 study)	⊕⊕⊖⊖ low[1,3]	SMD 0.08 (－0.43 to 0.59)
治疗结束后 4 周便秘评分差值 Follow－up: mean 4 weeks		The mean 治疗结束后 4 周便秘评分差值 in the intervention groups was 0.84 standard deviations higher (0.2 to 1.49 higher)		41 (1 study)	⊕⊕⊖⊖ low[1,3]	SMD 0.84 (0.2 to 1.49)
治疗结束后 12 周便秘评分差值 Follow－up: mean 4 weeks		The mean 治疗结束后 12 周便秘评分差值 in the intervention groups was 0.62 standard deviations higher (0.01 lower to 1.25 higher)		41 (1 study)	⊕⊕⊖⊖ low[1,3]	SMD 0.62 (－0.01 to 1.25)
治疗结束后 6 个月便秘评分差值 Follow－up: mean 4 weeks		The mean 治疗结束后 6 个月便秘评分差值 in the intervention groups was 0.32 standard deviations higher (0.3 lower to 0.93 higher)		41 (1 study)	⊕⊕⊖⊖ low[1,3]	SMD 0.32 (－0.3 to 0.93)
治疗 1 周满意度评价 Follow－up: mean 4 weeks		The mean 治疗 1 周满意度评价 in the intervention groups was 0.55 standard deviations lower (1.06 to 0.05 lower)		71 (1 study)	⊕⊕⊖⊖ low[1,3]	SMD －0.55 (－1.06 to －0.05)
治疗 2 周满意度评价 Follow－up: mean 4 weeks		The mean 治疗 2 周满意度评价 in the intervention groups was 0.33 standard deviations lower (0.83 lower to 0.17 higher)		71 (1 study)	⊕⊕⊖⊖ low[1,3]	SMD －0.33 (－0.83 to 0.17)
治疗 3 周满意度评价 Follow－up: mean 4 weeks		The mean 治疗 3 周满意度评价 in the intervention groups was 0.59 standard deviations lower (1.09 to 0.08 lower)		71 (1 study)	⊕⊕⊖⊖ low[1,3]	SMD －0.59 (－1.09 to －0.08)

续表

Outcomes	Illustrative comparative risks* (95% CI)		Relative effect (95% CI)	No of Participants (studies)	Quality of the evidence (GRADE)	Comments
	Assumed risk — Control	Corresponding risk — 电针 VS 电针				
治疗4周满意度评价 Follow – up: mean 4 weeks		The mean 治疗4周满意度评价 in the intervention groups was 0.91 standard deviations lower (1.43 to 0.39 lower)		71 (1 study)	⊕⊕⊕⊖ low[1,3]	SMD −0.91 (−1.43 to −0.39)
治疗前后焦患自评量表 SAS 差值 Follow – up: mean 4 weeks		The mean 治疗前后焦患自评量表 SAS 差值 in the intervention groups was 0.29 standard deviations lower (0.8 lower to 0.22 higher)		60 (1 study)	⊕⊕⊕⊖ low[3]	SMD −0.29 (−0.8 to 0.22)
治疗前后抑郁自评量表 SDS 差值 Follow – up: mean 4 weeks		The mean 治疗前后抑郁自评量表 SDS 差值 in the intervention groups was 0.14 standard deviations higher (0.37 lower to 0.65 higher)		60 (1 study)	⊕⊕⊕⊖ low[1,3]	SMD 0.14 (−0.37 to 0.65)
治疗前后症状自评量表 SCL – 90 阳性项目数差值 Follow – up: mean 4 weeks		The mean 治疗前后症状自评量表 SCL – 90 阳性项目数差值 in the intervention groups was 0.1 standard deviations higher (0.41 lower to 0.6 higher)		60 (1 study)	⊕⊕⊕⊖ low[1,3]	SMD 0.1 (−0.41 to 0.6)
总有效率	Study population 783 per 1000 Medium risk population 783 per 1000	924 per 1000 (760 to 1000) 924 per 1000 (760 to 1000)	RR 1.18 (0.97 to 1.44)	120 (2)		
总有效率 – 深刺天枢 VS 浅刺天枢 revman Follow – up: mean 4 weeks	Study population 733 per 1000 Medium risk population 733 per 1000	968 per 1000 (770 to 1000) 968 per 1000 (770 to 1000)	RR 1.32 (1.05 to 1.65)	60 (1 study)	⊕⊕⊕⊖ low[1,3]	
总有效率 – 低频电针 VS 高频电针 revman Follow – up: mean 4 weeks	Study population 833 per 1000 Medium risk population 833 per 1000	900 per 1000 (733 to 1000) 900 per 1000 (733 to 1000)	RR 1.08 (0.88 to 1.32)	60 (1 study)	⊕⊕⊖⊖ low[3]	

续表

Outcomes	Illustrative comparative risks* (95% CI)		Relative effect (95% CI)	No of Participants (studies)	Quality of the evidence (GRADE)	Comments
	Assumed risk Control	Corresponding risk 电针 VS 电针				
治疗前后结肠传输时间差值 Follow－up：mean 4 weeks		The mean 治疗前后结肠传输时间差值 in the intervention groups was 0.31 standard deviations higher (0.51 lower to 1.12 higher)		29 (1 study)	⊕⊕⊕⊝ moderate[1]	SMD 0.31 (−0.51 to 1.12)
治疗1周排便费力程度评分差值 Follow－up：mean 4 weeks		The mean 治疗1周排便费力程度评分差值 in the intervention groups was 0.23 standard deviations higher (0.28 lower to 0.74 higher)		131 (2 studies)	⊕⊕⊕⊝ moderate[3]	SMD 0.23 (−0.28 to 0.74)
治疗1周排便费力程度评分差值 － 深刺天枢 VS 浅刺天枢 Follow－up：mean 4 weeks		The mean 治疗1周排便费力程度评分差值 － 深刺天枢 VS 浅刺天枢 in the intervention groups was 0.23 standard deviations higher (0.28 lower to 0.74 higher)		131 (2 studies)		SMD 0.23 (−0.28 to 0.74)
治疗2周排便费力程度评分差值 Follow－up：mean 4 weeks		The mean 治疗2周排便费力程度评分差值 in the intervention groups was 0.15 standard deviations higher (0.2 lower to 0.51 higher)		131 (2 studies)	⊕⊕⊕⊝ moderate[3]	SMD 0.15 (−0.2 to 0.51)
治疗4周结束排便费力程度差值 Follow－up：mean 4 weeks		The mean 治疗4周结束排便费力程度差值 in the intervention groups was 0.36 standard deviations higher (0.07 to 0.66 higher)		191 (3 studies)		SMD 0.36 (0.07 to 0.66)
治疗4周结束排便费力程度差值 － 深刺天枢 VS 浅刺天枢 Follow－up：mean 4 weeks		The mean 治疗4周结束排便费力程度差值 － 深刺天枢 VS 浅刺天枢 in the intervention groups was 0.51 standard deviations higher (0.15 to 0.87 higher)		131 (2 studies)	⊕⊕⊕⊝ moderate[3]	SMD 0.51 (0.15 to 0.87)
治疗4周结束排便费力程度差值 － 低频电针 VS 高频电针 Follow－up：mean 4 weeks		The mean 治疗4周结束排便费力程度差值 － 低频电针 VS 高频电针 in the intervention groups was 0.06 standard deviations higher (0.44 lower to 0.57 higher)		60 (1 study)	⊕⊕⊝⊝ low[1,3]	SMD 0.06 (−0.44 to 0.57)
治疗结束12周排便费力程度评分差值 Follow－up：mean 4 weeks		The mean 治疗结束12周排便费力程度评分差值 in the intervention groups was 1.01 standard deviations higher (0.59 to 1.42 higher)		101 (2 studies)	⊕⊕⊕⊝ moderate[3]	SMD 1.01 (0.59 to 1.42)
治疗结束24周排便费力程度评分差值 Follow－up：mean 4 months		The mean 治疗结束24周排便费力程度评分差值 in the intervention groups was 0.87 standard deviations higher (0.46 to 1.28 higher)		101 (2 studies)	⊕⊕⊕⊝ moderate[3]	SMD 0.87 (0.46 to 1.28)

续表

Outcomes	Illustrative comparative risks* (95% CI)		Relative effect (95% CI)	No of Participants (studies)	Quality of the evidence (GRADE)	Comments
	Assumed risk Control	Corresponding risk 电针 VS 电针				
治疗4周结束后排便不尽感差值		The mean 治疗4周结束后排便不尽感差值 in the intervention groups was 0.37 standard deviations higher (0.18 lower to 0.93 higher)		191 (3 studies)		SMD 0.37 (−0.18 to 0.93)
治疗4周结束后排便不尽感差值 – 深刺天枢VS浅刺天枢 Follow－up: mean 4 weeks		The mean 治疗4周结束后排便不尽感差值 – 深刺天枢VS浅刺天枢 in the intervention groups was 0.56 standard deviations higher (0.19 lower to 1.31 higher)		131 (2 studies)	⊕⊕⊕⊖ low[2,3]	SMD 0.56 (−0.19 to 1.31)
治疗4周结束后排便不尽感差值 – 低频电针VS高频电针 Follow－up: mean 4 weeks		The mean 治疗4周结束后排便不尽感差值 – 低频电针VS高频电针 in the intervention groups was 0.01 standard deviations higher (0.5 lower to 0.52 higher)		60 (1 study)	⊕⊕⊕⊖ low[1,3]	SMD 0.01 (−0.5 to 0.52)
治疗结束后12周排便不尽感差值 Follow－up: mean 4 weeks		The mean 治疗结束后12周排便不尽感差值 in the intervention groups was 1.31 standard deviations higher (0.74 to 1.87 higher)		60 (1 study)	⊕⊕⊕⊖ low[1,3]	SMD 1.31 (0.74 to 1.87)
治疗结束后24周排便不尽感差值 Follow－up: mean 4 weeks		The mean 治疗结束后24周排便不尽感差值 in the intervention groups was 1.38 standard deviations higher (0.82 to 1.95 higher)		60 (1 study)	⊕⊕⊕⊖ low[1,3]	SMD 1.38 (0.82 to 1.95)
治疗4周大便质地差值 Follow－up: mean 4 weeks		The mean 治疗4周大便质地差值 in the intervention groups was 0.28 standard deviations higher (0.08 lower to 0.63 higher)		131 (2 studies)	⊕⊕⊕⊕ moderate[3]	SMD 0.28 (−0.08 to 0.63)
治疗后24周大便质地差值 Follow－up: mean 4 weeks		The mean 治疗后24周大便质地差值 in the intervention groups was 0.57 standard deviations higher (0.06 to 1.09 higher)		60 (1 study)	⊕⊕⊕⊖ low[1,3]	SMD 0.57 (0.06 to 1.09)
治疗4周结束排便频率频率评分差值 Follow－up: mean 4 weeks		The mean 治疗4周结束排便频率频率评分差值 in the intervention groups was 0.42 standard deviations higher (0.09 lower to 0.94 higher)		60 (1 study)	⊕⊕⊕⊕ moderate[1]	SMD 0.42 (−0.09 to 0.94)
治疗结束后12周排便频率评分差值 Follow－up: mean 4 weeks		The mean 治疗结束后12周排便频率频率评分差值 in the intervention groups was 1.04 standard deviations higher (0.38 to 1.69 higher)		41 (1 study)	⊕⊕⊕⊕ moderate[1]	SMD 1.04 (0.38 to 1.69)

续表

Outcomes	Illustrative comparative risks* (95% CI)		Relative effect (95% CI)	No of Participants (studies)	Quality of the evidence (GRADE)	Comments
	Assumed risk Control	Corresponding risk 电针 VS 电针				
治疗结束后6个月排便频率 率评分 率评分差值 Follow－up: mean 4 weeks		The mean 治疗结束后6个月排便频率率评分 差值 in the intervention groups was 0.87 standard deviations higher (0.22 to 1.51 higher)		41 (1 study)	⊕⊕⊕⊖ moderate[1]	SMD 0.87 (0.22 to 1.51)

* The basis for the assumed risk (e.g. the median control group risk across studies) is provided in footnotes. The corresponding risk (and its 95% confidence interval) is based on the assumed risk in the comparison group and the relative effect of the intervention (and its 95% CI).

CI: Confidence interval; RR: Risk ratio;

GRADE Working Group grades of evidence

High quality: Further research is very unlikely to change our confidence in the estimate of effect.

Moderate quality: Further research is likely to have an important impact on our confidence in the estimate of effect and may change the estimate.

Low quality: Further research is very likely to have an important impact on our confidence in the estimate of effect and is likely to change the estimate.

Very low quality: We are very uncertain about the estimate.

1 只有一篇文章纳入。
2 异质性。
3 主观指标。

电针 VS 药物 for 慢性便秘

Patient or population: patients with 慢性便秘
Settings:
Intervention: 电针 VS 药物

Outcomes	Illustrative comparative risks* (95% CI)		Relative effect (95% CI)	No of Participants (studies)	Quality of the evidence (GRADE)	Comments
	Assumed risk — Control	Corresponding risk — 电针 VS 药物				
治疗4周排便次数差值		The mean 治疗4周排便次数值 in the intervention groups was 0.13 standard deviations lower (0.58 lower to 0.32 higher)		344 (3 studies)	⊕⊕⊕⊕ high	SMD −0.13 (−0.58 to 0.32)
治疗4周排便次数差值 – 深刺天枢 VS 药物 Follow-up: mean 4 weeks		The mean 治疗4周排便次数值 – 深刺天枢 VS 药物 0.24 standard deviations higher (0.05 lower to 0.54 higher)		208 (3 studies)	⊕⊕⊕⊕ high	SMD 0.24 (−0.05 to 0.54)
治疗4周排便次数差值 – 常规刺天枢 VS 药物 Follow-up: mean 4 weeks		The mean 治疗4周排便次数值 – 常规刺天枢 VS 药物 0.16 standard deviations lower (0.73 lower to 0.41 higher)		49 (1 study)	⊕⊕⊕⊖ moderate[1]	SMD −0.16 (−0.73 to 0.41)
治疗4周排便次数差值 – 浅刺天枢 VS 药物 Follow-up: mean 4 weeks		The mean 治疗4周排便次数值 – 浅刺天枢 VS 药物 0.73 standard deviations lower (1.85 lower to 0.39 higher)		87 (2 studies)	⊕⊕⊖⊖ low[2,3]	SMD −0.73 (−1.85 to 0.39)
治疗2周总有效率 revman Follow-up: mean 4 weeks	Study population; 200 per 1000; Medium risk population 200 per 1000	766 per 1000 (364 to 1000); 766 per 1000 (364 to 1000)	RR 3.83 (1.82 to 8.05)	60 (1 study)	⊕⊕⊖⊖ low[1,4]	
治疗2周CCS评分差值 Follow-up: mean 2 weeks		The mean 治疗2周CCS评分差值 in the intervention groups was 0.61 standard deviations higher (0.09 to 1.13 higher)		60 (1 study)	⊕⊕⊖⊖ low[1,4]	SMD 0.61 (0.09 to 1.13)

Outcomes	Illustrative comparative risks* (95% CI)		Relative effect (95% CI)	No of Participants (studies)	Quality of the evidence (GRADE)	Comments
	Assumed risk Control	Corresponding risk 电针 VS 药物				
治疗 2 周结束后 6 个月总有效率 revman Follow－up: mean 26 weeks	Study population		RR 11.23 (1.61 to 78.06)	41 (1 study)	⊕⊕⊝⊝ low[1,4]	
	53 per 1000	595 per 1000 (85 to 1000)				
	Medium risk population					
	53 per 1000	595 per 1000 (85 to 1000)				
治疗 2 周结束后 6 个月 CCS 评分差值 Follow－up: mean 26 weeks	The mean 治疗 2 周结束后 6 个月 CCS 评分差值 in the intervention groups was 1.31 standard deviations higher (0.63 to 2 higher)			41 (1 study)	⊕⊕⊝⊝ low[1,4]	SMD 1.31 (0.63 to 2)
治疗 2 周 CTT 差值 Follow－up: mean 2 weeks	The mean 治疗 2 周 CTT 差值 in the intervention groups was 1.17 standard deviations higher (0.62 to 1.72 higher)			60 (1 study)	⊕⊕⊕⊝ moderate[1]	SMD 1.17 (0.62 to 1.72)
治疗 4 周 CCS 评分差值	The mean 治疗 4 周 CCS 评分差值 in the intervention groups was 0.61 standard deviations higher (0.13 to 1.08 higher)			427 (4 studies)		SMD 0.61 (0.13 to 1.08)
治疗 4 周 CCS 评分差值 － 深刺天枢 VS 药物 Follow－up: mean 4 weeks	The mean 治疗 4 周 CCS 评分差值 － 深刺天枢 VS 药物 in the intervention groups was 0.94 standard deviations higher (0.38 to 1.51 higher)			251 (4 studies)	⊕⊕⊝⊝ low[2,4]	SMD 0.94 (0.38 to 1.51)
治疗 4 周 CCS 评分差值 － 常规刺天枢 VS 药物 Follow－up: mean 4 weeks	The mean 治疗 4 周 CCS 评分差值 － 常规刺天枢 VS 药物 in the intervention groups was 0.17 standard deviations lower (0.84 lower to 0.51 higher)			89 (2 studies)	⊕⊕⊕⊝ moderate[4]	SMD －0.17 (－0.84 to 0.51)
治疗 4 周 CCS 评分差值 － 浅刺天枢 VS 药物 Follow－up: mean 4 weeks	The mean 治疗 4 周 CCS 评分差值 － 浅刺天枢 VS 药物 in the intervention groups was 0.71 standard deviations higher (0.22 to 1.64 higher)			87 (2 studies)	⊕⊕⊝⊝ low[2,4]	SMD 0.71 (－0.22 to 1.64)
治疗 4 周结束后 12 周 CCS 评分差值	The mean 治疗 4 周结束后 12 周 CCS 评分差值 in the intervention groups was 0.41 standard deviations higher (0.2 lower to 1.02 higher)			83 (1 study)	See comment	SMD 0.41 (－0.2 to 1.02)

续表

Outcomes	Illustrative comparative risks* (95% CI)		Relative effect (95% CI)	No of Participants (studies)	Quality of the evidence (GRADE)	Comments
	Assumed risk — Control	Corresponding risk — 电针 VS 药物				
治疗 4 周结束后 12 周 CCS 评分差值 – 深刺天枢 VS 药物 Follow – up: mean 16 weeks		The mean 治疗 4 周结束后 12 周 CCS 评分差值 – 深刺天枢 VS 药物 in the intervention groups was 0.72 standard deviations higher (0.1 to 1.34 higher)		43 (1 study)	⊕⊖⊖⊖ very low[1,4,5]	SMD 0.72 (0.1 to 1.34)
治疗 4 周结束后 12 周 CCS 评分差值 – 常规刺天枢 VS 药物 Follow – up: mean 16 weeks		The mean 治疗 4 周结束后 12 周 CCS 评分差值 – 常规刺天枢 VS 药物 in the intervention groups was 0.1 standard deviations higher (0.52 lower to 0.72 higher)		40 (1 study)	⊕⊖⊖⊖ very low[1,4,5]	SMD 0.1 (-0.52 to 0.72)
治疗 4 周结束后 6 个月 CCS 评分差值		The mean 治疗 4 周结束后 6 个月 CCS 评分差值 in the intervention groups was 0.21 standard deviations higher (0.22 lower to 0.64 higher)		83 (1)	See comment	SMD 0.21 (-0.22 to 0.64)
治疗 4 周结束后 6 个月 CCS 评分差值 – 深刺天枢 VS 药物 Follow – up: mean 28 weeks		The mean 治疗 4 周结束后 6 个月 CCS 评分差值 – 深刺天枢 VS 药物 in the intervention groups was 0.36 standard deviations higher (0.24 lower to 0.97 higher)		43 (1 study)	⊕⊖⊖⊖ very low[1,4,5]	SMD 0.36 (-0.24 to 0.97)
治疗 4 周结束后 6 个月 CCS 评分差值 – 常规刺天枢 VS 药物 Follow – up: mean 28 weeks		The mean 治疗 4 周结束后 6 个月 CCS 评分差值 – 常规刺天枢 VS 药物 in the intervention groups was 0.05 standard deviations higher (0.57 lower to 0.67 higher)		40 (1 study)	⊕⊖⊖⊖ very low[1,4,5]	SMD 0.05 (-0.57 to 0.67)
治疗 4 周结束后 4 周排便频率评分差值		The mean 治疗 4 周结束后 4 周排便频率评分差值 in the intervention groups was 0.12 standard deviations lower (1.54 lower to 1.3 higher)		83 (1 study)	See comment	SMD -0.12 (-1.54 to 1.3)
治疗 4 周结束后 4 周排便频率评分差值 – 深刺天枢 VS 药物 Follow – up: mean 8 weeks		The mean 治疗 4 周结束后 4 周排便频率评分差值 – 深刺天枢 VS 药物 in the intervention groups was 0.6 standard deviations higher (0.02 lower to 1.21 higher)		43 (1 study)	⊕⊕⊖⊖ low[1,5]	SMD 0.6 (-0.02 to 1.21)
治疗 4 周结束后 4 周排便频率评分差值 – 常规刺天枢 VS 药物 Follow – up: mean 8 weeks		The mean 治疗 4 周结束后 4 周排便频率评分差值 – 常规刺天枢 VS 药物 in the intervention groups was 0.85 standard deviations lower (1.5 to 0.2 lower)		40 (1 study)	⊕⊕⊖⊖ low[1,5]	SMD -0.85 (-1.5 to -0.2)

续表

Outcomes	Illustrative comparative risks* (95% CI)		Relative effect (95% CI)	No of Participants (studies)	Quality of the evidence (GRADE)	Comments
	Assumed risk Control	Corresponding risk 电针 VS 药物				
治疗 4 周结束后 12 周排便频率评分差值		The mean 治疗 4 周结束后 12 周排便频率评分值 in the intervention groups was 0.15 standard deviations lower (1.16 lower to 0.87 higher)		83 (1 study)	See comment	SMD −0.15 (−1.16 to 0.87)
治疗 4 周结束后 12 周排便频率评分差值 − 深刺天枢 VS 药物 Follow-up: mean 16 weeks		The mean 治疗 4 周结束后 12 周排便频率评分值 − 深刺天枢 VS 药物 in the intervention groups was 0.37 standard deviations higher (0.24 lower to 0.97 higher)		43 (1 study)	⊕⊕⊖⊖ low[1,5]	SMD 0.37 (−0.24 to 0.97)
治疗 4 周结束后 12 周排便频率评分差值 VS 药物 Follow-up: mean 16 weeks		The mean 治疗 4 周结束后 12 周排便频率评分值 − 常规刺天枢 VS 药物 in the intervention groups was 0.67 standard deviations lower (1.31 to 0.03 lower)		40 (1 study)	⊕⊕⊖⊖ low[1,5]	SMD −0.67 (−1.31 to −0.03)
治疗 4 周结束后 6 个月排便率评分差值		The mean 治疗 4 周结束后 6 个月排便频评分值 in the intervention groups was 0.14 standard deviations lower (0.97 lower to 0.68 higher)		83 (1 study)	See comment	SMD −0.14 (−0.97 to 0.68)
治疗 4 周结束后 6 个月排便率评分差值 − 深刺天枢 VS 药物 Follow-up: mean 28 weeks		The mean 治疗 4 周结束后 6 个月排便频评分值 − 深刺天枢 VS 药物 in the intervention groups was 0.27 standard deviations higher (0.33 lower to 0.87 higher)		43 (1 study)	⊕⊕⊖⊖ low[1,5]	SMD 0.27 (−0.33 to 0.87)
治疗 4 周结束后 6 个月排便率评分差值 − 常规刺天枢 VS 药物 Follow-up: mean 28 weeks		The mean 治疗 4 周结束后 6 个月排便频评分值 − 常规刺天枢 VS 药物 in the intervention groups was 0.57 standard deviations lower (1.21 lower to 0.06 higher)		40 (1 study)	⊕⊕⊖⊖ low[1,5]	SMD −0.57 (−1.21 to 0.06)
治疗 4 周后排便频率评分差值		The mean 治疗 4 周后排便频率评分差值 in the intervention groups was 0.03 standard deviations higher (0.35 lower to 0.4 higher)		129 (1 study)	See comment	SMD 0.03 (−0.35 to 0.4)
治疗 4 周后排便频率评分差值 − 深刺天枢 VS 药物 Follow-up: mean 4 weeks		The mean 治疗 4 周后排便频率评分差值 − 深刺天枢 VS 药物 in the intervention groups was 0.17 standard deviations higher (0.33 lower to 0.67 higher)		80 (1 study)	⊕⊕⊕⊖ moderate[1]	SMD 0.17 (−0.33 to 0.67)

续表

Outcomes	Illustrative comparative risks* (95% CI)		Relative effect (95% CI)	No of Participants (studies)	Quality of the evidence (GRADE)	Comments
	Assumed risk — Control	Corresponding risk — 电针 VS 药物				
治疗 4 周后排便频率评分差值 - 常规刺天枢 VS 药物 Follow-up: mean 4 weeks		The mean 治疗 4 周后排便频率评分差值 - 常规刺天枢 VS 药物 in the intervention groups was 0.15 standard deviations lower (0.72 lower to 0.42 higher)		49 (1 study)	⊕⊕⊕⊖ moderate[1]	SMD −0.15 (−0.72 to 0.42)
治疗 4 周排便费力程度评分差值		The mean 治疗 4 周排便费力程度评分差值 in the intervention groups was 0.59 standard deviations higher (0.06 lower to 1.24 higher)		248 (2 studies)		SMD 0.59 (−0.06 to 1.24)
治疗 4 周排便费力程度评分差值 - 深刺天枢 VS 药物 Follow-up: mean 4 weeks		The mean 治疗 4 周排便费力程度评分差值 - 深刺天枢 VS 药物 in the intervention groups was 0.73 standard deviations higher (0.48 lower to 1.95 higher)		152 (2 studies)	⊕⊖⊖⊖ very low[2,3,4]	SMD 0.73 (−0.48 to 1.95)
治疗 4 周排便费力程度评分差值 - 常规刺天枢 VS 药物 Follow-up: mean 4 weeks		The mean 治疗 4 周排便费力程度评分差值 - 常规刺天枢 VS 药物 in the intervention groups was 0.02 standard deviations lower (0.58 lower to 0.55 higher)		49 (1 study)	⊕⊕⊖⊖ low[1,4]	SMD −0.02 (−0.58 to 0.55)
治疗 4 周排便费力程度评分差值 - 浅刺天枢 VS 药物 Follow-up: mean 4 weeks		The mean 治疗 4 周排便费力程度评分差值 - 浅刺天枢 VS 药物 in the intervention groups was 0.92 standard deviations higher (0.32 to 1.53 higher)		47 (1 study)	⊕⊕⊖⊖ low[1,4]	SMD 0.92 (0.32 to 1.53)
治疗 4 周结束后 4 周排便费力程度评分差值		The mean 治疗 4 周结束后 4 周排便费力程度评分差值 in the intervention groups was 0.2 standard deviations higher (0.88 lower to 1.29 higher)		83 (1 study)	See comment	SMD 0.2 (−0.88 to 1.29)
治疗 4 周结束后 4 周排便费力程度评分差值 - 深刺天枢 VS 药物 Follow-up: mean 8 weeks		The mean 治疗 4 周结束后 4 周排便费力程度评分差值 - 深刺天枢 VS 药物 in the intervention groups was 0.75 standard deviations higher (0.13 to 1.37 higher)		43 (1 study)	⊕⊕⊖⊖ low[1,4]	SMD 0.75 (0.13 to 1.37)
治疗 4 周结束后 4 周排便费力程度评分差值 - 常规刺天枢 VS 药物 Follow-up: mean 8 weeks		The mean 治疗 4 周结束后 4 周排便费力程度评分差值 - 常规刺天枢 VS 药物 in the intervention groups was 0.35 standard deviations lower (0.98 lower to 0.27 higher)		40 (1 study)	⊕⊕⊖⊖ low[1,4]	SMD −0.35 (−0.98 to 0.27)
治疗 4 周结束后 12 周排便费力程度评分差值 Follow-up: mean 4 weeks		The mean 治疗 4 周结束后 12 周排便费力程度评分差值 in the intervention groups was 0.29 standard deviations lower (1.46 lower to 0.87 higher)		83 (1 study)	⊕⊕⊖⊖ low[1,4]	SMD −0.29 (−1.46 to 0.87)

续表

Outcomes	Illustrative comparative risks* (95% CI)		Relative effect (95% CI)	No of Participants (studies)	Quality of the evidence (GRADE)	Comments
	Assumed risk Control	Corresponding risk 电针 VS 药物				
治疗 4 周结束后 12 周排便费力程度评分差值 - 深刺天枢 VS 药物 Follow - up: mean 16 weeks		The mean 治疗 4 周结束后 12 周排便费力程度评分差值 - 深刺天枢 VS 药物 in the intervention groups was 0.29 standard deviations higher (0.31 lower to 0.89 higher)		43 (1 study)	⊕⊕⊖⊖ low[1,4]	SMD 0.29 (-0.31 to 0.89)
治疗 4 周结束后 12 周排便费力程度评分差值 VS 药物 Follow - up: mean 16 weeks		The mean 治疗 4 周结束后 12 周排便费力程度评分差值 - 常规刺天枢 VS 药物 in the intervention groups was 0.89 standard deviations lower (1.55 to 0.24 lower)		40 (1 study)	⊕⊕⊖⊖ low[1,5]	SMD -0.89 (-1.55 to -0.24)
治疗 4 周结束后 6 个月排便费力程度评分差值		The mean 治疗 4 周结束后 6 个月排便费力程度评分差值 in the intervention groups was 0 standard deviations higher (0.65 lower to 0.64 higher)		83 (1 study)	See comment	SMD 0 (-0.65 to 0.64)
治疗 4 周结束后 6 个月排便费力程度评分差值 - 深刺天枢 VS 药物 Follow - up: mean 28 weeks		The mean 治疗 4 周结束后 6 个月排便费力程度评分差值 - 深刺天枢 VS 药物 in the intervention groups was 0.32 standard deviations higher (0.28 lower to 0.92 higher)		43 (1 study)	⊕⊕⊖⊖ low[1,4]	SMD 0.32 (-0.28 to 0.92)
治疗 4 周结束后 6 个月排便费力程度评分差值 - 常规刺天枢 VS 药物 Follow - up: mean 28 weeks		The mean 治疗 4 周结束后 6 个月排便费力程度评分差值 - 常规刺天枢 VS 药物 in the intervention groups was 0.34 standard deviations lower (0.97 lower to 0.28 higher)		40 (1 study)	⊕⊕⊖⊖ low[1,4]	SMD -0.34 (-0.97 to 0.28)
治疗 4 周排便时间评分差值		The mean 治疗 4 周排便时间评分差值 in the intervention groups was 0.22 standard deviations higher (0.15 lower to 0.6 higher)		129 (1 study)	See comment	SMD 0.22 (-0.15 to 0.6)
治疗 4 周排便时间评分差值 - 深刺天枢 VS 药物 Follow - up: mean 4 weeks		The mean 治疗 4 周排便时间评分差值 - 深刺天枢 VS 药物 in the intervention groups was 0.39 standard deviations higher (0.12 lower to 0.89 higher)		80 (1 study)	⊕⊕⊕⊖ moderate[1]	SMD 0.39 (-0.12 to 0.89)
治疗 4 周排便时间评分差值 - 常规刺天枢 VS 药物 Follow - up: mean 4 weeks		The mean 治疗 4 周排便时间评分差值 - 常规刺天枢 VS 药物 in the intervention groups was 0.02 standard deviations higher (0.55 lower to 0.58 higher)		49 (1 study)	⊕⊕⊕⊖ moderate[1]	SMD 0.02 (-0.55 to 0.58)

续表

Outcomes	Illustrative comparative risks* (95% CI)		Relative effect (95% CI)	No of Participants (studies)	Quality of the evidence (GRADE)	Comments
	Assumed risk Control	Corresponding risk 电针 VS 药物				
治疗 4 周结束后 4 周排便时间评分差值		The mean 治疗 4 周结束后 4 周排便时间评分差值 in the intervention groups was 0.22 standard deviations higher (0.25 lower to 0.69 higher)		83 (1 study)	See comment	SMD 0.22 (−0.25 to 0.69)
治疗 4 周结束后 4 周排便时间评分差值 － 深刺天枢 VS 药物 Follow－up: mean 8 weeks		The mean 治疗 4 周结束后 4 周排便时间评分差值 － 深刺天枢 VS 药物 in the intervention groups was 0.46 standard deviations higher (0.15 lower to 1.07 higher)		43 (1 study)	⊕⊕⊕⊝ moderate[1]	SMD 0.46 (−0.15 to 1.07)
治疗 4 周结束后 4 周排便时间评分差值 － 常规刺天枢 VS 药物 Follow－up: mean 8 weeks		The mean 治疗 4 周结束后 4 周排便时间评分差值 － 常规刺天枢 VS 药物 in the intervention groups was 0.02 standard deviations lower (0.64 lower to 0.6 higher)		40 (1 study)	⊕⊕⊕⊝ moderate[1]	SMD −0.02 (−0.64 to 0.6)
治疗 4 周结束后 12 周排便时间评分差值		The mean 治疗 4 周结束后 12 周排便时间评分差值 in the intervention groups was 0.12 standard deviations higher (0.31 lower to 0.56 higher)		83 (1 study)	See comment	SMD 0.12 (−0.31 to 0.56)
治疗 4 周结束后 12 周排便时间评分差值 － 深刺天枢 VS 药物 Follow－up: mean 16 weeks		The mean 治疗 4 周结束后 12 周排便时间评分差值 － 深刺天枢 VS 药物 in the intervention groups was 0.27 standard deviations higher (0.33 lower to 0.87 higher)		43 (1 study)	⊕⊕⊕⊝ moderate[1]	SMD 0.27 (−0.33 to 0.87)
治疗 4 周结束后 12 周排便时间评分差值 － 常规刺天枢 VS 药物 Follow－up: mean 16 weeks		The mean 治疗 4 周结束后 12 周排便时间评分差值 － 常规刺天枢 VS 药物 in the intervention groups was 0.03 standard deviations lower (0.65 lower to 0.59 higher)		40 (1 study)	⊕⊕⊕⊝ moderate[1]	SMD −0.03 (−0.65 to 0.59)
治疗 4 周结束后 6 个月排便时间评分差值		The mean 治疗 4 周结束后 6 个月排便时间评分差值 in the intervention groups was 0.02 standard deviations lower (0.45 lower to 0.41 higher)		83 (1 study)	See comment	SMD −0.02 (−0.45 to 0.41)
治疗 4 周结束后 6 个月排便时间评分差值 － 深刺天枢 VS 药物 Follow－up: mean 28 weeks		The mean 治疗 4 周结束后 6 个月排便时间评分差值 － 深刺天枢 VS 药物 in the intervention groups was 0.02 standard deviations higher (0.58 lower to 0.62 higher)		43 (1 study)	⊕⊕⊕⊝ moderate[1]	SMD 0.02 (−0.58 to 0.62)

续表

Outcomes	Illustrative comparative risks* (95% CI)		Relative effect (95% CI)	No of Participants (studies)	Quality of the evidence (GRADE)	Comments
	Assumed risk Control	Corresponding risk 电针 VS 药物				
治疗4周结束后6个月排便时间评分间差值 VS 药物 Follow－up: mean 28 weeks		The mean 治疗4周结束后6个月排便时间评分间差值 － 常规刺天枢 VS 药物 in the intervention groups was 0.07 standard deviations lower (0.69 lower to 0.55 higher)		40 (1 study)	⊕⊕⊕⊖ moderate[1]	SMD －0.07 (－0.69 to 0.55)
治疗4周后CTT时间差值		The mean 治疗4周后CTT时间差值 in the intervention groups was 0.1 standard deviations higher (0.27 lower to 0.48 higher)		129 (1 study)	See comment	SMD 0.1 (－0.27 to 0.48)
治疗4周后CTT时间差值 － 深刺天枢 VS 药物 Follow－up: mean 4 days		The mean 治疗4周后CTT时间差值 － 深刺天枢 VS 药物 in the intervention groups was 0.15 standard deviations higher (0.34 lower to 0.65 higher)		80 (1 study)	⊕⊕⊕⊖ moderate[1]	SMD 0.15 (－0.34 to 0.65)
治疗4周后CTT时间差值 － 常规刺天枢 VS 药物 Follow－up: mean 4 weeks		The mean 治疗4周后CTT时间差值 － 常规刺天枢 VS 药物 in the intervention groups was 0.04 standard deviations higher (0.53 lower to 0.6 higher)		49 (1 study)	⊕⊕⊕⊖ moderate[1]	SMD 0.04 (－0.53 to 0.6)
首次排便时间		The mean 首次排便时间 in the intervention groups was 0.29 standard deviations lower (1.32 lower to 0.75 higher)		129 (1 study)	See comment	SMD －0.29 (－1.32 to 0.75)
首次排便时间 － 深刺天枢 VS 药物 Follow－up: mean 4 weeks		The mean 首次排便时间 － 深刺天枢 VS 药物 in the intervention groups was 0.81 standard deviations lower (1.32 to 0.29 lower)		80 (1 study)	⊕⊕⊕⊖ moderate[1]	SMD －0.81 (－1.32 to －0.29)
首次排便时间 － 常规刺天枢 VS 药物 Follow－up: mean 4 weeks		The mean 首次排便时间 － 常规刺天枢 VS 药物 in the intervention groups was 0.25 standard deviations higher (0.32 lower to 0.82 higher)		49 (1 study)	⊕⊕⊕⊖ moderate[1]	SMD 0.25 (－0.32 to 0.82)
治疗4周结束后4周排便次数差值		The mean 治疗4周结束后4周排便次数差值 in the intervention groups was 0.33 standard deviations lower (1.66 lower to 0.99 higher)		118 (1 study)	See comment	SMD －0.33 (－1.66 to 0.99)
治疗4周结束后4周排便次数差值 － 深刺天枢 VS 药物 Follow－up: mean 8 weeks		The mean 治疗4周结束后4周排便次数差值 － 深刺天枢 VS 药物 in the intervention groups was 0.33 standard deviations higher (0.17 lower to 0.83 higher)		71 (1 study)	⊕⊕⊕⊖ moderate[1]	SMD 0.33 (－0.17 to 0.83)

Outcomes	Illustrative comparative risks* (95% CI)		Relative effect (95% CI)	No of Participants (studies)	Quality of the evidence (GRADE)	Comments
	Assumed risk Control	Corresponding risk 电针 VS 药物				
治疗 4 周结束后 4 周排便次数差值 - 浅刺天枢 VS 药物 Follow – up: mean 8 weeks		The mean 治疗 4 周结束后 4 周排便次数差值 - 浅刺天枢 VS 药物 in the intervention groups was 1.02 standard deviations lower (1.63 to 0.41 lower)		47 (1 study)	⊕⊕⊕⊝ moderate[1]	SMD - 1.02 (- 1.63 to - 0.41)
治疗 4 周结束后 12 周排便次数差值 Follow – up: mean 12 weeks		The mean 治疗 4 周结束后 12 周排便次数差值 in the intervention groups was 0 standard deviations higher (0.89 lower to 0.89 higher)		118 (1 study)	See comment	SMD 0 (- 0.89 to 0.89)
治疗 4 周结束后 12 周排便次数差值 - 深刺天枢 VS 药物 Follow – up: mean 16 weeks		The mean 治疗 4 周结束后 12 周排便次数差值 - 深刺天枢 VS 药物 in the intervention groups was 0.44 standard deviations higher (0.06 lower to 0.94 higher)		71 (1 study)	⊕⊕⊕⊝ moderate[1]	SMD 0.44 (- 0.06 to 0.94)
治疗 4 周结束后 12 周排便次数差值 - 浅刺天枢 VS 药物 Follow – up: mean 16 weeks		The mean 治疗 4 周结束后 12 周排便次数差值 - 浅刺天枢 VS 药物 in the intervention groups was 0.47 standard deviations lower (1.05 lower to 0.11 higher)		47 (1 study)	⊕⊕⊕⊝ moderate[1]	SMD - 0.47 (- 1.05 to 0.11)
治疗 4 周结束后 6 个月排便次数差值		The mean 治疗 4 周结束后 6 个月排便次数差值 in the intervention groups was 0.17 standard deviations higher (1.22 lower to 1.57 higher)		118 (1 study)	See comment	SMD 0.17 (- 1.22 to 1.57)
治疗 4 周结束后 6 个月排便次数差值 - 深刺天枢 VS 药物 Follow – up: mean 28 weeks		The mean 治疗 4 周结束后 6 个月排便次数差值 - 深刺天枢 VS 药物 in the intervention groups was 0.88 standard deviations higher (0.36 to 1.4 higher)		71 (1 study)	⊕⊕⊕⊝ moderate[1]	SMD 0.88 (0.36 to 1.4)
治疗 4 周结束后 6 个月排便次数差值 - 浅刺天枢 VS 药物 Follow – up: mean 4 weeks		The mean 治疗 4 周结束后 6 个月排便次数差值 - 浅刺天枢 VS 药物 in the intervention groups was 0.54 standard deviations lower (1.13 lower to 0.04 higher)		47 (1 study)	⊕⊕⊕⊝ moderate[1]	SMD - 0.54 (- 1.13 to 0.04)
治疗 4 周大便不尽感评分差值 Follow – up: mean 4 weeks		The mean 治疗 4 周大便不尽感评分差值 in the intervention groups was 0.67 standard deviations higher (0.3 to 1.03 higher)		248 (2 studies)	⊕⊕⊕⊝ moderate[4]	SMD 0.67 (0.3 to 1.03)
治疗 4 周大便不尽感评分差值 - 深刺天枢 VS 药物 Follow – up: mean 4 weeks		The mean 治疗 4 周大便不尽感评分差值 - 深刺天枢 VS 药物 in the intervention groups was 0.72 standard deviations higher (0.11 to 1.33 higher)		152 (2 studies)	⊕⊕⊕⊝ moderate[4]	SMD 0.72 (0.11 to 1.33)

续表

Outcomes	Illustrative comparative risks* (95% CI)		Relative effect (95% CI)	No of Participants (studies)	Quality of the evidence (GRADE)	Comments
	Assumed risk Control	Corresponding risk 电针 VS 药物				
治疗 4 周大便不尽感评分差值 - 浅刺天枢 VS 药物 Follow-up: mean 4 weeks		The mean 治疗 4 周大便不尽感评分差值 - 浅刺天枢 VS 药物 0.94 standard deviations higher in the intervention groups was (0.33 to 1.54 higher)		47 (1 study)	⊕⊕⊖⊖ low[1,4]	SMD 0.94 (0.33 to 1.54)
治疗 4 周大便不尽感评分差值 - 常规刺天枢 VS 药物 Follow-up: mean 4 weeks		The mean 治疗 4 周大便不尽感评分差值 - 常规刺天枢 VS 药物 0.3 standard deviations higher in the intervention groups was (0.27 lower to 0.87 higher)		49 (1 study)	⊕⊕⊖⊖ low[1,4]	SMD 0.3 (-0.27 to 0.87)
治疗 4 周大便质地评分差值		The mean 治疗 4 周大便质地评分差值 in the intervention groups was 0.38 standard deviations higher (0.01 to 0.76 higher)		119 (1 study)	See comment	SMD 0.38 (0.01 to 0.76)
治疗 4 周大便质地评分差值 - 深刺天枢 VS 药物 Follow-up: mean 4 weeks		The mean 治疗 4 周大便质地评分差值 - 深刺天枢 VS 药物 0.47 standard deviations higher in the intervention groups was (0.02 lower to 0.97 higher)		72 (1 study)	⊕⊕⊖⊖ low[1,4]	SMD 0.47 (-0.02 to 0.97)
治疗 4 周大便质地评分差值 - 浅刺天枢 VS 药物 Follow-up: mean 4 weeks		The mean 治疗 4 周大便质地评分差值 - 浅刺天枢 VS 药物 0.26 standard deviations higher in the intervention groups was (0.32 lower to 0.83 higher)		47 (1 study)	⊕⊕⊖⊖ low[1,4]	SMD 0.26 (-0.32 to 0.83)
治疗 4 周满意度评分差值		The mean 治疗 4 周满意度评分差值 1.75 standard deviations lower in the intervention groups was (2.48 to 1.03 lower)		119 (1 study)	See comment	SMD -1.75 (-2.48 to -1.03)
治疗 4 周满意度评分差值 - 深刺天枢 VS 药物 Follow-up: mean 4 weeks		The mean 治疗 4 周满意度评分差值 - 深刺天枢 VS 药物 2.12 standard deviations lower in the intervention groups was (2.72 to 1.51 lower)		72 (1 study)	⊕⊕⊖⊖ low[1,4]	SMD -2.12 (-2.72 to -1.51)
治疗 4 周满意度评分差值 - 浅刺天枢 VS 药物 Follow-up: mean 4 weeks		The mean 治疗 4 周满意度评分差值 - 浅刺天枢 VS 药物 1.37 standard deviations lower in the intervention groups was (2.02 to 0.73 lower)		47 (1 study)	⊕⊕⊖⊖ low[1,4]	SMD -1.37 (-2.02 to -0.73)

续表

Outcomes	Illustrative comparative risks* (95% CI)		Relative effect (95% CI)	No of Participants (studies)	Quality of the evidence (GRADE)	Comments
	Assumed risk Control	Corresponding risk 电针 VS 药物				

* The basis for the assumed risk (e. g. the median control group risk across studies) is provided in footnotes. The corresponding risk (and its 95% confidence interval) is based on the assumed risk in the comparison group and the relative effect of the intervention (and its 95% CI).
CI: Confidence interval; RR: Risk ratio;

GRADE Working Group grades of evidence
High quality: Further research is very unlikely to change our confidence in the estimate of effect.
Moderate quality: Further research is likely to have an important impact on our confidence in the estimate of effect and may change the estimate.
Low quality: Further research is very likely to have an important impact on our confidence in the estimate of effect and is likely to change the estimate.
Very low quality: We are very uncertain about the estimate.

1 只有一篇文献纳入。
2 异质性较大。
3 未来发表文献有可能逆转结果。
4 主观性指标。
5 样本量小。

115

手针＋生物反馈 compared to 生物反馈 for 慢性便秘

Patient or population: patients with 慢性便秘
Settings:
Intervention: 手针＋生物反馈
Comparison: 生物反馈

Outcomes	Illustrative comparative risks * (95% CI)		Relative effect (95% CI)	No of Participants (studies)	Quality of the evidence (GRADE)	Comments
	Assumed risk 生物反馈	Corresponding risk 手针＋生物反馈				
治疗 3 周结束每周大便次数差值 Follow－up: mean 3 weeks		The mean 治疗 3 周结束每周大便次数差值 in the intervention groups was 0.39 standard deviations lower (0 to 0.2 higher)		45 (1 study)	⊕⊖⊖⊖ very low[1,2,3]	
治疗结束 1 个月后大便次数差值 Follow－up: mean 7 weeks		The mean 治疗结束 1 个月后大便次数差值 in the intervention groups was 0.88 standard deviations higher (0.27 to 1.5 higher)		45 (1 study)	⊕⊖⊖⊖ very low[1,2,3]	
治疗 3 周结束排便困难积分 Follow－up: mean 3 weeks		The mean 治疗 3 周结束排便困难积分 in the intervention groups was 0.21 standard deviations lower (0.71 lower to 0.47 higher)		45 (1 study)	⊕⊖⊖⊖ very low[1,2,3,4]	
治疗结束 1 个月后排便困难积分 Follow－up: mean 7 weeks		The mean 治疗结束 1 个月后排便困难积分 in the intervention groups was 0.79 standard deviations higher (0.17 to 1.4 higher)		45 (1 study)	⊕⊖⊖⊖ very low[1,2,3,4]	
治疗 3 周结束大便性状积分差值 Follow－up: mean 3 weeks		The mean 治疗 3 周结束大便性状积分差值 in the intervention groups was 0.46 standard deviations higher (0.14 lower to 1.06 higher)		45 (1 study)	⊕⊖⊖⊖ very low[1,2,3,4]	
治疗 3 周结束肛门直肠测压各项指标差值 Follow－up: mean 3 weeks		The mean 治疗 3 周结束肛门直肠测压各项指标差值 in the intervention groups was 0 higher (0 to 0 higher)		45 (1 study)	⊕⊖⊖⊖ very low[1,2,3]	
治疗结束 1 个月肛门直肠测压各指标差值 Follow－up: mean 7 weeks		The mean 治疗结束 1 个月肛门直肠测压各指标差值 in the intervention groups was 0 higher (0 to 0 higher)		45 (1 study)	⊕⊖⊖⊖ very low[1,2,3]	

续表

Outcomes	Illustrative comparative risks * (95% CI)		Relative effect (95% CI)	No of Participants (studies)	Quality of the evidence (GRADE)	Comments
	Assumed risk 生物反馈	Corresponding risk 手针 + 生物反馈				
治疗结束 1 个月大便性状积分差值 Follow – up: mean 7 weeks		The mean 治疗结束 1 个月大便性状积分差值 in the intervention groups was 1.15 standard deviations higher (0.52 to 1.79 higher)		45 (1 study)	$\oplus\ominus\ominus\ominus$ very low[1,2,3,4]	

* The basis for the assumed risk (e. g. the median control group risk across studies) is provided in footnotes. The corresponding risk (and its 95% confidence interval) is based on the assumed risk in the comparison group and the relative effect of the intervention (and its 95% CI) .

CI: Confidence interval;

GRADE Working Group grades of evidence

High quality: Further research is very unlikely to change our confidence in the estimate of effect.

Moderate quality: Further research is likely to have an important impact on our confidence in the estimate of effect and may change the estimate.

Low quality: Further research is very likely to have an important impact on our confidence in the estimate of effect and is likely to change the estimate.

Very low quality: We are very uncertain about the estimate.

1 非随机对照。

2 样本量小。

3 只有一篇文献纳入。

4 主观指标。

电针 + 电脑中频治疗仪 compared to 电脑中频治疗仪 for 慢性便秘

Patient or population: patients with 慢性便秘
Settings:
Intervention: 电针 + 电脑中频治疗仪
Comparison: 电脑中频治疗仪

Outcomes	Illustrative comparative risks* (95% CI)		Relative effect (95% CI)	No of Participants (studies)	Quality of the evidence (GRADE)	Comments
	Assumed risk	Corresponding risk				
	电脑中频治疗仪	电针 + 电脑中频治疗仪				
	Study population					
显效率 Follow – up: mean 2 weeks	600 per 1000	774 per 1000 (546 to 1000)	RR 1.29 (0.91 to 1.83)	61 (1 study)	⊕⊝⊝⊝ very low[1,2,3]	
	Medium risk population					
	600 per 1000	774 per 1000 (546 to 1000)				

* The basis for the assumed risk (e. g. the median control group risk across studies) is provided in footnotes. The corresponding risk (and its 95% confidence interval) is based on the assumed risk in the comparison group and the relative effect of the intervention (and its 95% CI).
CI: Confidence interval; RR: Risk ratio;

GRADE Working Group grades of evidence
High quality: Further research is very unlikely to change our confidence in the estimate of effect.
Moderate quality: Further research is likely to have an important impact on our confidence in the estimate of effect and may change the estimate.
Low quality: Further research is very likely to have an important impact on our confidence in the estimate of effect and is likely to change the estimate.
Very low quality: We are very uncertain about the estimate.

1 非随机对照。
2 主观指标。
3 只有一篇文献纳入。

两组穴位交替针刺 for 慢性功能性便秘

Patient or population: patients with 慢性功能性便秘
Settings:
Intervention: 两组穴位交替针刺

Outcomes	Illustrative comparative risks * (95% CI)		Relative effect (95% CI)	No of Participants (studies)	Quality of the evidence (GRADE)	Comments
	Assumed risk	Corresponding risk				
	Control	两组穴位交替针刺				
生活质量积分 Follow – up: mean 20 days		The mean 生活质量积分 in the intervention groups was 0 higher (0 to 0 higher)		90 (1 study[4])	⊕⊝⊝⊝ very low[1,2,3]	case series; mean 0 higher (0 to 0 higher)
症状积分 Follow – up: mean 20 days		The mean 症状积分 in the intervention groups was 0 higher (0 to 0 higher)		90 (1 study[4])	⊕⊝⊝⊝ very low[1,2,3]	case series; mean 0 higher (0 to 0 higher)
每次排便时间 Follow – up: mean 20 days		The mean 每次排便时间 in the intervention groups was 0 higher (0 to 0 higher)		90 (1 study[4])	⊕⊝⊝⊝ very low[1,3]	case series; mean 0 higher (0 to 0 higher)
治疗结束时有效率 Follow – up: mean 20 days			RR 0 (0 to 0)	90 (1 study[4])	⊕⊝⊝⊝ very low[2,3,4]	case series; 72 events in 0 subjects
治疗结束后 1 个月有效率 Follow – up: mean 20 days			RR 0 (0 to 0)	90 (1 study[4])	⊕⊝⊝⊝ very low[2,3,4]	case series; 70 events in 0 subjects
治疗结束后 3 个月有效率 Follow – up: mean 20 days			RR 0 (0 to 0)	90 (1 study[4])	⊕⊝⊝⊝ very low[2,3,4]	case series; 62 events in 0 subjects

* The basis for the assumed risk (e. g. the median control group risk across studies) is provided in footnotes. The corresponding risk (and its 95% confidence interval) is based on the assumed risk in the comparison group and the relative effect of the intervention (and its 95% CI).
CI: Confidence interval; RR: Risk ratio;

GRADE Working Group grades of evidence
High quality: Further research is very unlikely to change our confidence in the estimate of effect.
Moderate quality: Further research is likely to have an important impact on our confidence in the estimate of effect and may change the estimate.
Low quality: Further research is very likely to have an important impact on our confidence in the estimate of effect and is likely to change the estimate.
Very low quality: We are very uncertain about the estimate.

1 观察性研究。
2 主观指标。
3 只有一篇文献纳入。
4 Case Series.

音频电疗 + 针刺 compared to 针刺 for 老年习惯性便秘

Patient or population: patients with 老年习惯性便秘
Settings:
Intervention: 音频电疗 + 针刺
Comparison: 针刺

Outcomes	Illustrative comparative risks * (95% CI)		Relative effect (95% CI)	No of Participants (studies)	Quality of the evidence (GRADE)	Comments
	Assumed risk	Corresponding risk				
	针刺	音频电疗 + 针刺				
有效率 Follow – up: mean 45 days	Medium risk population		OR 0 (0 to 0)	162 (1 study)	⊕⊝⊝⊝ very low[1,2,3]	

* The basis for the assumed risk (e. g. the median control group risk across studies) is provided in footnotes. The corresponding risk (and its 95% confidence interval) is based on the assumed risk in the comparison group and the relative effect of the intervention (and its 95% CI).
CI: Confidence interval; OR: Odds ratio;

GRADE Working Group grades of evidence
High quality: Further research is very unlikely to change our confidence in the estimate of effect.
Moderate quality: Further research is likely to have an important impact on our confidence in the estimate of effect and may change the estimate.
Low quality: Further research is very likely to have an important impact on our confidence in the estimate of effect and is likely to change the estimate.
Very low quality: We are very uncertain about the estimate.

1 Case – control.
2 主观性指标。
3 只纳入一篇文献。

针刺 + 腹部推拿 compared to 五仁润肠丸 for 老年性虚证便秘

Patient or population: patients with 老年性虚证型便秘
Settings:
Intervention: 针刺 + 腹部推拿
Comparison: 五仁润肠丸

Outcomes	Illustrative comparative risks* (95% CI)		Relative effect (95% CI)	No of Participants (studies)	Quality of the evidence (GRADE)	Comments
	Assumed risk	Corresponding risk				
	五仁润肠丸	针刺 + 腹部推拿				
	Study population					
		967 per 1000 (747 to 1000)				
总有效率 Follow – up: mean 20 days	667 per 1000		RR 1.45 (1.12 to 1.88)	60 (1 study)	⊕◯◯◯ very low[1,2,3]	
	Medium risk population					
	667 per 1000	967 per 1000 (747 to 1000)				

* The basis for the assumed risk (e. g. the median control group risk across studies) is provided in footnotes. The corresponding risk (and its 95% confidence interval) is based on the assumed risk in the comparison group and the relative effect of the intervention (and its 95% CI).
CI: Confidence interval; RR: Risk ratio;

GRADE Working Group grades of evidence
High quality: Further research is very unlikely to change our confidence in the estimate of effect.
Moderate quality: Further research is likely to have an important impact on our confidence in the estimate of effect and may change the estimate.
Low quality: Further research is very likely to have an important impact on our confidence in the estimate of effect and is likely to change the estimate.
Very low quality: We are very uncertain about the estimate.

1 假随机。
2 主观性指标。
3 只有一篇文献纳入。

水针＋益气润肠汤 compared to 麻仁丸 for 老年习惯性便秘

Patient or population: patients with 老年习惯性便秘
Settings:
Intervention: 水针＋益气润肠汤
Comparison: 麻仁丸

Outcomes	Illustrative comparative risks* (95% CI)		Relative effect (95% CI)	No of Participants (studies)	Quality of the evidence (GRADE)	Comments
	Assumed risk	Corresponding risk				
	麻仁丸	水针＋益气润肠汤				
	Study population					
有效率 Follow－up: mean 40 days	1000 per 1000	1000 per 1000 (990 to 1000)	RR 1 (0.99 to 1.01)	376 (1 study)	⊕⊕⊕⊖ very low[1,2,3]	
	Medium risk population					
	1000 per 1000	1000 per 1000 (990 to 1000)				
便秘消失时间 Follow－up: mean 40 days		The mean 便秘消失时间 in the intervention groups was 2.98 standard deviations lower (3.28 to 2.69 lower)		376 (1 study)	⊕⊕⊕⊖ very low[1,3]	
便秘复发时间 Follow－up: mean 40 days		The mean 便秘复发时间 in the intervention groups was 44.68 standard deviations higher (41.46 to 47.9 higher)		376 (1 study)	⊕⊕⊕⊖ very low[1,3]	

* The basis for the assumed risk (e. g. the median control group risk across studies) is provided in footnotes. The corresponding risk (and its 95% confidence interval) is based on the assumed risk in the comparison group and the relative effect of the intervention (and its 95% CI) .
CI: Confidence interval; RR: Risk ratio;

GRADE Working Group grades of evidence
High quality: Further research is very unlikely to change our confidence in the estimate of effect.
Moderate quality: Further research is likely to have an important impact on our confidence in the estimate of effect and may change the estimate.
Low quality: Further research is very likely to have an important impact on our confidence in the estimate of effect and is likely to change the estimate.
Very low quality: We are very uncertain about the estimate.

1 非随机对照试验。
2 主观性指标。
3 只有一篇文献纳入。

手针 for 糖尿病性便秘

Patient or population: patients with 糖尿病性便秘
Settings:
Intervention: 手针

Outcomes	Illustrative comparative risks* (95% CI)		Relative effect (95% CI)	No of Participants (studies)	Quality of the evidence (GRADE)	Comments
	Assumed risk Control	Corresponding risk 手针				
总有效率 Follow – up: mean 34 days			RR 0 (0 to 0)	30 (1 study[1])	⊕⊝⊝⊝ very low[1,2,3,4]	case series; 28 events in 0 subjects

* The basis for the assumed risk (e. g. the median control group risk across studies) is provided in footnotes. The corresponding risk (and its 95% confidence interval) is based on the assumed risk in the comparison group and the relative effect of the intervention (and its 95% CI).
CI: Confidence interval; RR: Risk ratio;

GRADE Working Group grades of evidence
High quality: Further research is very unlikely to change our confidence in the estimate of effect.
Moderate quality: Further research is likely to have an important impact on our confidence in the estimate of effect and may change the estimate.
Low quality: Further research is very likely to have an important impact on our confidence in the estimate of effect and is likely to change the estimate.
Very low quality: We are very uncertain about the estimate.

1 Case Series.
2 主观性指标。
3 样本量小。
4 只有一篇文献纳入。

深刺天枢 for 结肠慢转运型便秘

Patient or population: patients with 结肠慢转运型便秘
Settings:
Intervention: 深刺天枢

Outcomes	Illustrative comparative risks* (95% CI)		Relative effect (95% CI)	No of Participants (studies)	Quality of the evidence (GRADE)	Comments
	Assumed risk Control	Corresponding risk 深刺天枢				
30 例的 CCS 积分 Follow-up: mean 2 weeks		The mean 30 例的 CCS 积分 in the intervention groups was 0 higher (0 to 0 higher)		30 (1 study[1])	⊕⊝⊝⊝ very low[1,2,3,4]	case series; mean 0 higher (0 to 0 higher)
30 例的 CTT 结果 Follow-up: mean 2 weeks		The mean 30 例的 CTT 结果 in the intervention groups was 0 higher (0 to 0 higher)		30 (1 study[1])	⊕⊝⊝⊝ very low[1,3,4]	case series; mean 0 higher (0 to 0 higher)
30 例的 CCS 有效率 Follow-up: mean 2 weeks			RR 0 (0 to 0)	30 (1 study[1])	⊕⊝⊝⊝ very low[1,2,3,4]	case series; 23 events in 0 subjects
15 例的 CCS 积分 Follow-up: mean 2 weeks		The mean 15 例的 CCS 积分 in the intervention groups was 0 higher (0 to 0 higher)		15 (1 study[1])	⊕⊝⊝⊝ very low[1,2,3,4]	case series; 0 events in 0 subjects
15 例的 CCS 有效率 Follow-up: mean 2 weeks			RR 0 (0 to 0)	15 (1 study[1])	⊕⊝⊝⊝ very low[1,2,3,4]	case series; 14 events in 0 subjects
15 例的 CTT 结果 Follow-up: mean 2 weeks		The mean 15 例的 CTT 结果 in the intervention groups was 0 higher (0 to 0 higher)		15 (1 study[1])	⊕⊝⊝⊝ very low[1,2,3,4]	case series; mean 0 higher (0 to 0 higher)
15 例的 CCT 有效率 Follow-up: mean 2 weeks			RR 0 (0 to 0)	15 (1 study[1])	⊕⊝⊝⊝ very low[1,2,3,4]	case series; 12 events in 0 subjects

续表

* The basis for the assumed risk (e.g. the median control group risk across studies) is provided in footnotes. The corresponding risk (and its 95% confidence interval) is based on the assumed risk in the comparison group and the relative effect of the intervention (and its 95% CI).

CI: Confidence interval; RR: Risk ratio;

GRADE Working Group grades of evidence

High quality: Further research is very unlikely to change our confidence in the estimate of effect.

Moderate quality: Further research is likely to have an important impact on our confidence in the estimate of effect and may change the estimate.

Low quality: Further research is very likely to have an important impact on our confidence in the estimate of effect and is likely to change the estimate.

Very low quality: We are very uncertain about the estimate.

1 Case Series.

2 主观性指标。

3 样本量较小。

4 只有一篇文献纳入。

轮流电针两组穴 for 慢传输型便秘

Patient or population: patients with 慢传输型便秘

Settings:

Intervention: 轮流电针两组穴

Outcomes	Illustrative comparative risks* (95% CI)		Relative effect (95% CI)	No of Participants (studies)	Quality of the evidence (GRADE)	Comments
	Assumed risk Control	Corresponding risk 轮流电针两组穴				
QOL 身体不适差值 Follow-up: mean 20 days	See comment	The mean QOL 身体不适差值 in the intervention groups was 0 higher (0 to 0 higher)		30 (1 study[1])	⊕⊖⊖⊖ very low[1,2,3,4]	case series; MD 0 higher (0 to 0 higher)
QOL 心理不适 Follow-up: mean 20 days	See comment	The mean QOL 心理不适 in the intervention groups was 0 higher (0 to 0 higher)		30 (1 study[1])	⊕⊖⊖⊖ very low[1,2,3,4]	case series; mean 0 higher (0 to 0 higher)
QOL 便秘相关的焦虑 Follow-up: mean 20 days	—	Study population	RR 0 (0 to 0)	0 (1 study[1])	See comment	case series; 0 events in 0 subjects
	See comment	See comment				
	—	Medium risk population				

续表

Outcomes	Illustrative comparative risks* (95% CI)		Relative effect (95% CI)	No of Participants (studies)	Quality of the evidence (GRADE)	Comments
	Assumed risk Control	Corresponding risk 轮流电针两组穴				
	Study population					
		-				
QOL 满意度 Follow – up: mean 20 days	See comment	See comment	RR 0 (0 to 0)	0 (1 study[1])	See comment	case series; 0 events in 0 subjects
	Medium risk population					
	-	-				
治疗结束有效率 Follow – up: mean 20 days			RR 0 (0 to 0)	30 (1 study[1])	⊕◯◯◯ very low[1,2,3,4]	case series; 22 events in 0 subjects
治疗结束 1 个月有效率 Follow – up: mean 1 months			RR 0 (0 to 0)	30 (1 study[1])	⊕◯◯◯ very low[1,2,3,4]	case series; 17 events in 0 subjects
治疗结束 3 个月有效率 Follow – up: mean 3 months			RR 0 (0 to 0)	30 (1 study[1])	⊕◯◯◯ very low[1,2,3,4]	case series; 15 events in 0 subjects

* The basis for the assumed risk (e. g. the median control group risk across studies) is provided in footnotes. The corresponding risk (and its 95% confidence interval) is based on the assumed risk in the comparison group and the relative effect of the intervention (and its 95% CI).
CI: Confidence interval; RR: Risk ratio;

GRADE Working Group grades of evidence
High quality: Further research is very unlikely to change our confidence in the estimate of effect.
Moderate quality: Further research is likely to have an important impact on our confidence in the estimate of effect and may change the estimate.
Low quality: Further research is very likely to have an important impact on our confidence in the estimate of effect and is likely to change the estimate.
Very low quality: We are very uncertain about the estimate.

1 Case Series.
2 主观性指标。
3 样本量小。
4 只纳入一篇文献。

润肠汤＋埋线 compared to 西沙必利片 for 慢传输型便秘

Patient or population: patients with 慢传输型便秘
Settings:
Intervention: 润肠汤＋埋线
Comparison: 西沙必利片

Outcomes	Illustrative comparative risks* (95% CI)		Relative effect (95% CI)	No of Participants (studies)	Quality of the evidence (GRADE)	Comments
	Assumed risk 西沙必利片	Corresponding risk 润肠汤＋埋线				
症状积分比较 Follow－up: mean 1 months		The mean 症状积分比较 in the intervention groups was 1.23 standard deviations higher (0.79 to 1.66 higher)		97 (1 study)	⊕⊙⊙⊙ very low[1,2,3]	

* The basis for the assumed risk (e. g. the median control group risk across studies) is provided in footnotes. The corresponding risk (and its 95% confidence interval) is based on the assumed risk in the comparison group and the relative effect of the intervention (and its 95% CI).
CI: Confidence interval;

GRADE Working Group grades of evidence
High quality: Further research is very unlikely to change our confidence in the estimate of effect.
Moderate quality: Further research is likely to have an important impact on our confidence in the estimate of effect and may change the estimate.
Low quality: Further research is very likely to have an important impact on our confidence in the estimate of effect and is likely to change the estimate.
Very low quality: We are very uncertain about the estimate.

1 非随机同期对照。
2 主观指标。
3 只有一篇文献纳入。

针灸 + 生物反馈 compared to 盆底肌训练 for 盆底松弛综合征型便秘

Patient or population: patients with 盆底松弛综合征便秘
Settings:
Intervention: 针灸 + 生物反馈
Comparison: 盆底肌训练

Outcomes	Illustrative comparative risks* (95% CI)		Relative effect (95% CI)	No of Participants (studies)	Quality of the evidence (GRADE)	Comments
	Assumed risk 盆底肌训练	Corresponding risk 针灸 + 生物反馈				
	Study population					
有效率 Follow – up: mean 20 days	200 per 1000	850 per 1000 (348 to 1000)	RR 4.25 (1.74 to 10.41)	40 (1 study)	⊕⊖⊖⊖ very low[1,2,3,4]	
	Medium risk population					
	200 per 1000	850 per 1000 (348 to 1000)				
PAC – QOL 评分 Follow – up: mean 20 days		The mean PAC – QOL 评分 in the intervention groups was 0.7 standard deviations higher (0.06 to 1.34 higher)		40 (1 study)	⊕⊖⊖⊖ very low[1,2,3,4]	

* The basis for the assumed risk (e. g. the median control group risk across studies) is provided in footnotes. The corresponding risk (and its 95% confidence interval) is based on the assumed risk in the comparison group and the relative effect of the intervention (and its 95% CI) .
CI: Confidence interval; RR: Risk ratio;

GRADE Working Group grades of evidence
High quality: Further research is very unlikely to change our confidence in the estimate of effect.
Moderate quality: Further research is likely to have an important impact on our confidence in the estimate of effect and may change the estimate.
Low quality: Further research is very likely to have an important impact on our confidence in the estimate of effect and is likely to change the estimate.
Very low quality: We are very uncertain about the estimate.

1 假 RCT。
2 主观性指标。
3 样本量小。
4 只纳入一篇文献。

穴位埋线 compared to 手针 for 慢性便秘

Patient or population: patients with 慢性便秘
Settings:
Intervention: 穴位埋线
Comparison: 手针

Outcomes	Illustrative comparative risks * (95% CI)		Relative effect (95% CI)	No of Participants (studies)	Quality of the evidence (GRADE)	Comments
	Assumed risk 手针	Corresponding risk 穴位埋线				
总有效率 revman Follow – up: mean 8 weeks	806 per 1000	943 per 1000 (830 to 1000)	RR 1.17 (1.03 to 1.33)	144 (1 study)	⊕⊖⊖⊖ very low[1,2,3]	

* The basis for the assumed risk (e. g. the median control group risk across studies) is provided in footnotes. The corresponding risk (and its 95% confidence interval) is based on the assumed risk in the comparison group and the relative effect of the intervention (and its 95% CI).
CI: Confidence interval; RR: Risk ratio;

GRADE Working Group grades of evidence
High quality: Further research is very unlikely to change our confidence in the estimate of effect.
Moderate quality: Further research is likely to have an important impact on our confidence in the estimate of effect and may change the estimate.
Low quality: Further research is very likely to have an important impact on our confidence in the estimate of effect and is likely to change the estimate.
Very low quality: We are very uncertain about the estimate.

1 分配隐藏及盲法存在缺陷。
2 主观性指标。
3 只纳入一个研究。

6 本《指南》推荐方案的形成过程

6.1 组建针灸治疗慢性便秘临床实践指南制定小组

6.1.1 人员组成

指南组汇集跨专业、多学科领域的专家、学者、研究人员、部分患者或护理人员，共同组成循证针灸临床实践指南（慢性便秘）委员会，委员会设立一名负责人，专项负责指南各委员会之间的协调、指南的进度把握、在中国针灸学会的监督下进行课题基金的调度、指南中期的回报、指南完成后的审核申报、指南后期的推广、宣传、发布、更新等事宜；设立一名秘书，负责会议召开通知、专家联络、培训协调、调配各委员会工作、问卷发放等事宜。本委员会由专家委员会、指南撰写委员会、患者及护理人员共同组成。每个分委会设置一名负责人。各成员均明确分工。

专家委员会由针灸临床、科研、消化科、中医文献学、临床流行病学、循证医学、医学统计学、医学计算机等领域的专家和学者组成，承担指南撰写委员会人员的培训工作。此外，对于确立并制定指南的框架，确立临床关键问题，制定文献检索范围、策略、方法，设计数据提取表格，制定针灸文献质量评估标准，确定推荐方案强度和等级，以及进行文献质量评价及治疗方案的推荐等工作起到重要作用，负责指导并协助指南撰写委员会人员完成指南撰写工作。

指南撰写委员会包括指南撰写、文献检索、数据提取及数据库录入人员。指南撰写人员经过培训后，在专家委员会的指导下展开指南编写工作，依据汇总后的医生及患者问卷的问题，筛选并确立临床关键问题；将评估后的文献根据临床研究疾病的特点（如疾病的分期、病情的严重程度）合并，治疗方案汇总，依据指南框架撰写。如在撰写过程中遇到问题或困难，通过指南委员会秘书向专家委员会提交问题以待解决。文献检索人员经过培训后，根据文献检索范围、策略、方法，针对不同类型的文献进行检索。数据人员根据数据提取表格提取文献数据。

6.1.2 人员分工

6.1.2.1 专家委员会

专家委员会包括针灸临床专家、神经内科专家、消化病学专家、流行病学及循证医学专家、统计学专家等，负责文献质量及证据等级评定，明确诊疗方法的推荐意见等。

6.1.2.2 委员会秘书

委员会秘书负责会议记录、各种资料的保留等。

6.1.2.3 编写委员会

编写委员会包括数据提取人员、文献检索人员、指南编写及翻译人员等。

6.1.2.4 患者及护理人员

患者及护理人员提供相关信息。

6.1.3 人员培训

在开始制定临床实践指南之前，需要对编写人员进行指南指定的一些基本知识及根据国际最新流行趋势的系统培训。

由于针灸学的特殊性，其强调从整体、动态、个体、功能的角度来研究人体的健康问题，所以针灸临床实践指南也有其特殊性，需对参与起草的人员进行有关的培训，明确目的，统一思路。

数据的提取、表格的填写、数据库的录入、文献质量评价、证据等级评定等也需要进行培训。

培训内容包括循证医学、指南方法学、医学统计学、临床流行病学、中医文献学、文献检索、数据挖掘等。

6.2 明确临床问题

6.2.1 医生及患者问卷的设计、反馈和汇总

为确立指南中的临床关键问题，由专家委员会成员设计医生及患者问卷，问卷涉及医生、患者临床上关心的针灸治疗慢性便秘的相关问题，如针灸治疗慢性便秘的近远期疗效、安全性、不良反应、

经济学分析、疗程等。临床医生及慢性便秘患者根据问卷提示回答问题。经委员会秘书汇总临床问题后，进行问题归类，提交指南撰写委员会并对临床问题进行筛选。

6.2.2 临床关键问题的筛选、确立

指南所覆盖的临床关键问题应遵循 PICO（patient intervention comparison and outcome）模型，即临床问题应包括目标人群、重要的干预措施及方法，干预措施间的比较，以及干预措施的临床疗效、危害和风险及对临床经济学的影响等。

依据 PICO 模型及众多的针灸方法，我们确立了共性问题、个性问题两类临床问题。①共性问题：讨论治疗慢性便秘的最佳操作方法、干预时机、激量、频次、疗程；不同病程时期、不同病情严重程度、不同年龄段患者的最佳针灸治疗方法；针灸对慢性便秘患者的早期确诊及避免误诊是否有帮助；针灸治疗慢性便秘的各种注意事项、并发症的预防及处理；慢性便秘患者的自我护理；针灸治疗慢性便秘患者的不良反应及禁忌证；患者对针灸干预措施的耐受度；针灸治疗的卫生经济学评价是否优于其他疗法。②个性问题：单纯针灸（电针、毫针、艾灸、腹针、头针）或配合其他疗法治疗慢性便秘的疗效、安全性、患者耐受情况、卫生经济学评价，以及不同治疗方法之间的疗效、安全性、不良反应、卫生经济学方面的比较；电针、毫针、艾灸、腹针、头针治疗慢性便秘的器具、仪器的最佳标准。

通过对上述问题反复推敲、研究，专家委员会成员推出筛选后的临床关键问题，即共性问题 8 个，个性问题 28 个。

6.3 文献检索

在进行文献检索之前，我们进行了文献的初步检索，了解针灸治疗慢性便秘临床文献的类别情况，随后经中医文献学专家、循证医学专家对文献进行分类。

6.3.1 制定文献检索策略

严格制定指南涉及有关证据的收集和合成过程，应采用系统的方法检索证据，文献检索应针对每个关键的问题。由于生物医学文献量非常大，单个资源（库）难以满足所需证据，单一的检索策略已不可能定位于检索范围广泛的证据资源。

6.3.2 提供检索策略的细节

指南应提供检索策略的细节，包括关键词的选用、检索的时间跨度和所使用的资源。至少应包括以下资源：Cochrane Library、EMBASE、MEDLINE、CBM、CMCC 数据库以及日韩相关数据库，因特网上重要的专业学会、协会和指南出版机构的网站，在研临床试验数据库或网站等。同时，检索相关古籍及专家经验，在有时间或可获得有关资源的情况下，配合手工检索。

6.4 文献证据评估标准的制定及评估

6.4.1 背景及目的

GRADE 系统是近年来由推荐分级的评估、制定与评价（GRADE）工作组的 80 余位国际专家研究和制定的最新评价系统，与以往的评价系统相比较，GRADE 系统有以下优势：①由一个具有广泛代表性的国际指南制定小组制定；②明确界定了证据质量和推荐强度；③清楚评价了不同治疗方案的重要结局；④对不同级别证据的升级与降级有明确、综合的标准；⑤从证据到推荐全程透明；⑥明确承认价值观和意愿；⑦就推荐意见的强弱，分别从临床医生、患者、政策制定者角度作了明确实用的诠释；⑧适用于制作系统评价、卫生技术评估及指南。

鉴于国际文献证据评估体系的发展和 GRADE 系统的优势特色，本《指南》决定采用 GRADE 系统作为文献证据评估的基本工具，并依据该系统制定本《指南》的文献证据质量评估标准。

6.4.2 制定文献质量评价标准的方法

从 2006 年起，BMJ 在其网站 bmj. com "稿约"中要求作者在投临床指南类文章时，最好按"推荐分级的评估、制定与评价"GRADE 系统对证据进行分级。迄今为止，GRADE 系统已被超过 25 个

组织广泛采纳，包括世界卫生组织、美国内科医师协会、美国胸科协会 UpToDate（一个在北美广泛使用的电子医书，www. uptodate.com）及 Cochrane 协作网。为达到透明和简化的目标，GRADE 系统将证据质量分为高、中、低、极低四级。证据质量及其定义如下：

高质量：进一步研究也不可能改变该疗效评估结果的可信度。

中等质量：进一步研究很可能影响该疗效评估结果的可信度，且可能改变该评估结果。

低质量：进一步研究极有可能影响该疗效评估结果的可信度，且该评估结果很可能改变。

极低质量：任何疗效评估结果都很不确定。

本指南组在上述评价系统的基础上，结合专家共识的方法，形成循证针灸临床实践指南的文献质量评价标准。

6.4.3 文献质量评价内容

本《指南》以国际最新的 GRADE（Grading of Recommendations Assessment，Development，and E-valuation）证据质量评价系统作为文献质量评价工具。

6.4.3.1 GRADE 将证据群的质量分为四类

GRADE 方法最终将证据群的质量分为高、中、低和极低四类。这四类质量各自的 GRADE 含义见下表，并将当前定义与之前的定义作了比较。之前的定义侧重证据等级对将来研究的意义（质量越低，则将来的研究越有可能改变我们对效应估计的信心及效应估计值本身）。之前定义的特征受到批评，我们认为是合理的，因为很多情况下我们不可能期待将来会有较高质量的证据。但我们也认为，当有理由相信将可获得新的有力证据时，之前的质量分级特征不失为是一种替代的方法。

证据四个等级的含义

质量等级	当前定义	早前定义
高	我们非常确信真实的效应值接近效应估计值	进一频研究非常不可能改变我们对效应估计值的确信程度
中	对效应估计值我们有中等程度的信心：真实值有可能接近估计值，但仍存在二者大不相同的可能性	进一步研究有可能对我们对效应估计值的确信程度造成重要影响，且可能改变该估计值
低	我们对效应估计值的确信程度有限：真实值可能与估计值大不相同	进一步研究很有可能对我们对效应估计值的确信程度造成重要影响，且可能改变该估计值
极低	我们对效应估计值几乎没有信心：真实值很可能与估计值大不相同	任何效应估计值都是非常不确定的

6.4.3.2 GRADE 文献质量评价的五个减分项和三个加分项

GRADE 所指的质量评价，是对所有研究每一重要结果的总体评价。评价证据质量之前，指南制定者应确定所有可能的重要结果，包括有益的、有害的及费用。然后，评价员才评价每一重要结果的证据质量。

GRADE 证据质量分级方法概要

研究设计	证据集群的初始质量	如果符合以下条件，降级	如果符合以下条件，升级	证据集群的质量等级
随机试验	高——→	偏倚风险 －1 严重 －2 非常严重 不一致性 －1 严重 －2 非常严重	效应量大 +1 大 +2 非常大 剂量反应 +1 梯度量效证据	高（4 个" +"：++++） 中（3 个" +"：+++ ○）

研究设计	证据集群的初始质量	如果符合以下条件，降级	如果符合以下条件，升级	证据集群的质量等级
观察性研究	低——→	间接性 -1 严重 -2 非常严重 不精确性 -1 严重 -2 非常严重 发表偏倚 -1 可能 -2 非常可能	所有可能的剩余混杂因素 +1 降低所展示的效应 +1 如未观察到效应，意味着是一种假效应	低（2个"+"：++○○） 极低（1个"+"：+○○○）

6.4.3.3　GRADE 将评估证据质量的过程与给出推荐建议的过程分开

推荐强度的判断不只依赖于证据质量，虽然相比于较低质量证据，较高质量证据更可能对应强推荐，但某特定质量等级的证据并不意味着特定强度的推荐，有时低或极低质量的证据仍可得出强推荐。

6.4.4　现代文献质量评价过程

三位经过规范化培训的评价员逐篇翻阅每篇文献（分为电子版与手工版文献），分别在广安门医院图书馆、军事医学院图书馆及协和医科大学图书馆进行。

制定针灸指南随机对照试验（RCT）文献偏倚风险电话确认 SOP，由专人针对入选的 RCT 进行逐篇确认。遴选在随机、对照、盲法、病例纳入排除标准、脱落病例处理等方面真正符合 RCT 特点的真 RCT。

由专门的 GRADE 评价员对文献进行综合评价。评价工具为 Review Manager 5.2 和 GRADE Profiler 3.2.2。

文献质量评价结果以 GRADE 证据概要表和结果总结表形式输出。其中，结果总结表用来汇总证据（以显示证据质量及每一重要结果的相对效应量和绝对效应量），证据概要表形式额外提供证据质量评价理由的详细信息。

6.5　制定推荐强度标准并形成推荐方案

作为国际最新的证据质量评价与分级系统，GRADE 系统简单明了地整合了证据质量和推荐强度的分级，方便专家、患者、临床医生及政策制定者使用。对证据质量和推荐强度详尽、明确地区分标准有助于指南和推荐的使用更加透明化。因此，本指南依据该系统制定的推荐强度标准形成针灸治疗慢性便秘的推荐方案。

6.5.1　证据分类合成

便秘可以是某些疾病的症状之一，也可以单独作为一种疾病存在。依据病因的不同，可分为功能性便秘与器质性便秘两类。根据临床表现和病理特点的不同，便秘又可分为慢传输型、出口梗阻型和混合型三个类型。便秘的分类与分型之间互有交叉。同时，年龄、性别、中医辨证分型对便秘的治疗效果也构成影响。

因此，推荐方案的形成应以病理分型为主线，结合其他要素形成推荐，条目尽量细化，以达到提纲挈领的目的。

6.5.2　推荐强度标准的制定

6.5.2.1　决定推荐强度的关键因素

决定推荐强度的关键因素有四个：第一个关键因素是在充分权衡不同治疗方案利弊基础上的利弊平衡；第二个关键因素是证据质量；第三个关键因素是患者价值观和意愿的不确定性或多变性；第四个关键因素是费用，成本比其他因素更易受时间、地理区域的影响而变化。

影响推荐强度的因素

影响因素	解释
利弊权衡	利弊之间的差距越大，越有可能被列为强推荐；利弊之间的差距越小，越有可能被列为弱推荐
证据质量	证据质量越高，越有可能被列为强推荐
价值观和意愿	价值观和意愿选择越多样化，或价值观和意愿选择不确定性越大，越有可能被列为弱推荐
成本（资源分配）	干预措施的成本越高（即消耗更多的资源），被列为强推荐的可能性越小

6.5.2.2 推荐强度的表达方法

GRADE 推荐强度提供了首选的符号描述法，同时也为喜欢使用数字和字母形式的机构提供了首选的数字/字母描述法。符号描述法更加直观，而且表示了支持和反对的方向，建议采用。

支持使用某项干预措施的强推荐↑ ↑ or 1；

支持使用某项干预措施的弱推荐↑ or 2；

反对使用某项干预措施的弱推荐↓ or 2；

反对使用某项干预措施的强推荐↓ ↓ or 1。

6.5.2.3 专家共识的方法

6.5.2.3.1 参与专家共识推荐意见的专家构成与组成

推荐专家组由 50 名以上正高职称人员组成，其中临床一线专家占 90% 以上，绝大多数为针灸专业人员。专家组由中国针灸学会标准化工作委员会负责遴选。

6.5.2.3.2 专家共识的方式

专家共识将采取会议或多轮专家问卷调查的形式。要求专家对每个推荐意见确定是否推荐，对推荐意见进行排序，并提出建议。同时，将专家共识的过程、结果，尤其是意见不一致之处均记录在案。

6.5.2.3.2.1 会议共识

要求 20 名以上的专家参会才可召开，采取无记名投票的方式取得推荐意见。

6.5.2.3.2.2 多轮专家问卷调查（德尔菲法）

将初步形成的推荐意见，以专家问卷的形式发送给专家，每轮专家至少 30 名以上。一般需要经过至少三轮专家问卷调查，才能形成推荐意见初稿。

专家共识的等级与标准

专家共识的等级	证据水平
A 级共识	符合三者之一：① 1 项针灸防治方案的高质量证据；② 1 项针灸防治方案的中等质量证据，并有古代文献证据和专家经验证据；③ 1 项针灸防治方案的中等质量证据，参与推荐的专家 70% 以上同意推荐
B 级共识	符合三者之一：① 1 项针灸防治方案的中等质量证据；② 2 项以上针灸防治方案的低质量证据，并有古代文献证据和专家经验证据；③ 2 项以上针灸防治方案的低质量证据，参与推荐的专家 50% ~70% 同意推荐
C 级共识	符合三者之一：① 2 项以上针灸防治方案的低质量证据；② 2 项以上针灸防治方案的极低质量证据，并有古代文献证据和专家经验证据；③ 2 项针灸防治方案的极低质量证据，参与推荐的专家 50% ~70% 同意推荐

6.5.3 推荐意见的形成

推荐方案的主要内容包括治疗原则、具体方案（包括取穴、操作、疗程）和推荐意见三部分，不同的疾病可以根据疾病的特点有所调整。由指南编写专家委员会对推荐意见逐条讨论，最终形成指南推荐意见。本指南将小组成员达成共识的方法及意见不一致之处，均记录在案。

7 本《指南》推荐方案征求意见稿

7.1 慢性功能性便秘针灸治疗推荐方案

7.1.1 未明确分型的慢性功能性便秘

对于未进行病理分型的慢性功能性便秘患者，推荐采用深刺天枢穴加电针疗法治疗。对于不能或不愿接受针刺治疗的慢性功能性便秘患者，推荐采用耳穴压丸疗法治疗。

7.1.2 结肠慢传输型便秘

推荐采用深刺天枢穴加电针疗法治疗结肠慢传输型便秘。对于不能或不愿接受针刺治疗的结肠慢传输型便秘患者，推荐采用热敏灸法治疗。

7.1.3 慢性功能性便秘（肠道气滞型）

推荐以电针支沟穴治疗慢性功能性便秘（肠道气滞型）。

7.1.4 老年慢性功能性便秘

推荐以"靳三针"中的肠三针、四神针、脑三针、足三针配合治疗老年慢性功能性便秘。

7.2 便秘型肠易激综合征针灸治疗推荐方案

在具备人员和门诊手术条件的医疗单位，在充分考虑患者意愿的前提下，推荐以指针配合穴位埋线疗法治疗便秘型肠易激综合征。

7.3 盆底失弛缓综合征针灸治疗推荐方案

推荐以毫针刺法结合生物反馈治疗盆底失弛缓综合征。推荐以深刺中髎、下髎穴治疗盆底失弛缓综合征。

7.4 糖尿病性便秘针灸治疗推荐方案

推荐以毫针刺法结合中药疗法治疗糖尿病性便秘。

8 专家意见征集过程、结果汇总及处理

本指南共进行了两轮专家意见的征集。

8.1 第一轮

第一轮在北京市范围内征求了同行业专家的意见，共收到9份反馈意见。原方案以病理分型为主线，结合其他要素形成推荐，条目尽量细化，以期达到提纲挈领的目的，形成分类＋分型＋辨证、分类＋分型、分类＋辨证、分型＋辨证、分类＋年龄、分类＋性别、单纯分类、单纯分型共8个条目。专家对于此种推荐意见形成方案进行了点评，建议根据临床研究的实际情况，删除过于繁复、临床指导意义不强的条目，根据专家意见，删除了分类＋分型＋辨证、分类＋分型，保留了其他6个条目。进一步考虑到便秘的发病、病情严重程度及治疗效果受到诸多因素的影响，不同体质的患者在便秘针灸治疗方面也应该区别对待，体现个体化原则，最终将推荐方案拟订为一般人群慢性便秘的针灸治疗和特定人群慢性便秘的针灸治疗两个方面。

8.2 第二轮

第二轮在全国范围内征求了针灸专家的意见，共收到11份反馈意见。各位专家针对治疗总则，分类、分型治疗中的10条推荐意见的条目、内容及文字描述，进行了精确的推敲，对某些个别条目的推荐等级进行了调整。根据GRADE系统决定推荐强度的四个关键因素，考虑老年便秘患者普遍病程较长，基础疾病多，心理耐受力差，药物、手术治疗等对此类患者不适合，针灸治疗对此类患者利弊差距大，且老年患者普遍对针灸疗法接受度高，时间宽裕，适合针灸治疗等因素，将推荐以"靳三针"中的肠三针、四神针、脑三针、足三针配合治疗老年慢性功能性便秘的推荐等级由弱推荐调

整为强推荐。

9　会议纪要

9.1　2013 年针灸临床实践指南项目审查会会议纪要

时间：2013 年 9 月 28 日。

地点：成都。

参会人员：国家中医药管理局、中国针灸学会的有关领导，以及全国针灸行业的科、教、研各方面共 26 名专家出席了会议，此外，还有 20 余名标准及指南起草单位的代表参加了会议。会议由中国针灸学会会长，全国针灸标准化技术委员会、中国针灸学会标准化工作委员会（以下简称"两针标委会"）主任委员刘保延主持，刘炜宏副主任委员、余曙光副主任委员分别担任 28 日上午和下午两个时间段的审查专家组组长。

会议内容：

国家中医药管理局政策法规与监督司查德忠司长到会并做了重要讲话。查司长在讲话中指出，标准化工作是国家中医药管理局法监司的工作重点，受到各方面的重视，局里已陆续出台一系列关于标准化工作的意义、规划及管理办法的文件以指导相关工作，同时已得到中央财政设中医标准化专款支持标准化项目。查司长鼓励针灸行业继续积极开展标准化工作，争取长久进展，他特别强调，要重视针灸标准体系和针灸标准化支撑体系的构建，要将针灸标准的制定与应用相结合，将标准的评价与应用相结合，要积极推进针灸标准化培训工作。在讲话最后，查司长提出了四点建议：一是要继续完善针灸标准化体系框架；二是要加强标准通则的制定；三是要围绕针灸临床实践来制定标准；四是要夯实针灸标准制定的基础。

中国针灸学会会长刘保延代表学会及两针标委会介绍了参加本次审查会的 2 项针灸国家标准、1 项针灸学会标准以及 15 项针灸临床实践指南项目的实施情况。在两针标委会的组织下，该 18 项标准（指南）的编制过程，严格遵循国家标准化管理委员会及中国针灸学会有关规定。目前，各项目组已对标准（指南）草案在全国范围内广泛征求意见，在今年 6 月份召开的两针标委会 2013 年年会上，该 18 项标准（指南）草案已通过初审。本次会议受国家中医药管理局委托，由两针标委会组织专家对标准（指南）送审稿进行审查。刘保延会长特别强调，临床实践指南是未来针灸标准化工作的重点，其性质更加贴近临床，其研制目的是为临床疗效和质量提供保障，所以，本次审订会上，针灸临床实践指南的评审重点是推荐方案的实用性。刘保延会长特请本次审查委员会专家严格把关，以确保标准（指南）的质量，他希望没有通过审查的项目起草单位能够做好修改和完善工作。

本次审查会对提交大会的 2 项针灸国家标准、1 项学会标准及 15 项针灸临床实践指南进行了审议，根据专家评审意见及专家投票情况得出评审结果：通过国家标准 1 项、学会标准 1 项、行业指南 6 项；建议修改后函审的行业指南 3 项；建议修改后会审的国家标准 1 项；未通过的行业指南 6 项。具体情况如下：

（1）审议通过的项目

专家审查委员会审查通过了由全国针灸标准化技术委员会起草的针灸国家标准《针灸临床治疗指南制定及评估规范》，由湖北中医药大学起草的中国针灸学会标准《针刀基本技术操作规范》，由中国中医科学院广安门医院起草的《慢性便秘针灸临床实践指南》和《腰痛针灸临床实践指南》，由北京中医药大学东直门医院起草的《原发性痛经针灸临床实践指南》，由成都中医药大学起草的《坐骨神经痛针灸临床实践指南》，由中国中医科学院针灸研究所起草的《失眠针灸临床实践指南》和《支气管哮喘（成人）针灸临床实践指南》。

（2）修改后函审的项目

由中国中医科学院针灸研究所起草的《肩周炎针灸临床实践指南》、由天津中医药大学起草的

《膝骨性关节炎针灸临床实践指南》以及由北京中医药大学东直门医院起草的《过敏性鼻炎针灸临床实践指南》3 项指南，建议按照评审意见修订后再行函审。

（3）修改后会审的项目

由南京中医药大学起草的针灸国家标准《针灸门诊服务规范》，建议按照评审意见修订后再行会审。

（4）未通过的项目

由安徽中医学院附属针灸医院起草的《神经根型颈椎病针灸临床实践指南》、由天津中医药大学起草的《慢性萎缩性胃炎针灸临床实践指南》、由南京中医药大学起草的《突发性耳聋针灸临床实践指南》和《单纯性肥胖病针灸临床实践指南》、由浙江中医药大学附属医院起草的《原发性三叉神经痛针灸临床实践指南》以及由陕西中医学院起草的《糖尿病周围神经病变针灸临床实践指南》6 项指南课题未通过审查。未通过审查的课题组按照评审意见继续修改和完善指南草案，由两针标委会秘书处另行安排验收审查。

最后，专家审查委员会提出，对于审议通过的标准，还需要对其内容及形式进行一致性修改，各标准起草单位应按照本次会议审查意见进行修改后，形成标准报批稿，上报两针标委会秘书处，经收集、整理、审核后，上报有关部门批准、发布。

《慢性便秘针灸临床实践指南》（送审稿）专家审查意见

2013 年 9 月 28 日，全国针灸标准化技术委员会、中国针灸学会标准化工作委员会在成都组织召开了"2013 年针灸标准及临床实践指南项目审查会"，会上审查了学会标准《慢性便秘针灸临床实践指南》（送审稿）。以刘炜宏为组长的 22 人专家组经过认真评议，形成如下意见：

本标准针对慢性便秘针灸临床实践，通过收集、整理慢性便秘针灸临床实践和科研的相关文献资料、调研分析、专家论证，以古今文献、临床实践为依据，详细规定了该指南简介、疾病概述、临床特点、诊断标准、治疗概况、针灸治疗、推荐方案、附件等方面内容，形成了慢性便秘针灸临床实践指南，并广泛征求专家意见，合理处理并分析相关意见，达成了共识。

专家组一致认为，本针灸临床实践指南的编写方法符合标准化的有关规定，资料完整，用语确切，格式规范；指南框架及内容系统实用，具有科学性和可行性；慢性便秘针灸临床治疗推荐方案合理，具备公认性和适用性；规定的针灸临床实践指南要求符合当前的科技水平和发展方向。

专家提出如下修订建议：

1. 有关推荐方案

（1）推荐方案中不应涉及针具品牌，推荐方案区分过细。

（2）建议增加辨证施治的内容，电针双侧支沟穴不妥，安全性差，不适合心脏病患者；天枢穴深刺也有安全问题，应用推荐依据。

（3）毫针粗细的描述应为毫米，不应该描述为 28 号，与长度一样，都用毫米。

（4）建议去掉中医辨证分型，不符合临床实际；西医诊断配针灸治疗，是否符合针灸临床实际？加大与临床实际的契合度，细化方案。

（5）进针时深度如何掌控？推荐的靳三针、四神针等可列入附录。

（6）针灸治疗前必须先行西医诊断，才能采用针灸治疗，而不是通过中医方法辨证分型。

（7）第 18 页"【3 - 5】"应规范写法。

2. 有关指南简介

（1）内容偏多，应简化；标点符号、文字错误较多。

（2）治疗人群中，中医证型和西医诊断夹杂，治疗思路和主线不清晰。

审查组同意该指南通过审查，建议根据专家意见修改后，以行业标准上报审批。

全国针灸标准化技术委员会
中国针灸学会标准化工作委员会
2013 年 9 月 28 日

附：《慢性便秘针灸临床实践指南》项目评审专家名单

序号	姓名	职称/职务	工作单位
1	刘炜宏	编审	中国中医科学院针灸所
2	文碧玲	教授	中国针灸学会
3	余曙光	副校长/研究员	成都中医药大学
4	郭 义	教授	天津中医药大学
5	杨 骏	院长/教授	安徽中医学院
6	赵京生	研究员	中国中医科学院针灸所
7	杨华元	教授	上海中医药大学
8	房繁恭	研究员	中国中医科学院针灸所
9	储浩然	主任医师	安徽省针灸医院
10	赵 宏	主任医师	中国中医科学院广安门医院
11	石 现	主任医师	解放军总医院针灸科
12	王富春	院长/教授	长春中医药大学针灸推拿学院
13	王麟鹏	主任医师	首都医科大学附属北京中医医院
14	贾春生	主任医师	河北医科大学中医学院
15	余晓阳	主任医师	重庆市中医院
16	高希言	教授	河南中医学院
17	常小荣	教授	湖南中医药大学
18	张洪涛	主任医师	甘肃省中医院
19	吕明庄	主任医师	贵州省贵阳医学院附属医院
20	王玲玲	院长/教授	南京中医药大学
21	宣丽华	主任医师	浙江中医药大学附属第一医院
22	翟 伟	教授	内蒙古医科大学中医学院

9.2 第二批针灸临床实践推荐方案专家论证会会议纪要

时间：2014 年 3 月 20 日。

地点：中国中医科学院 201 会议室。

参会成员：刘保延、武晓冬、刘志顺、王麟鹏、赵宏、6 个针灸临床实践指南课题组负责人及主要人员等。

会议议题：审查第二批针灸临床实践指南推荐方案；专家就指南推荐方案中的不足给予纠正和补充；讨论并统一针灸临床实践指南定稿的最终版式。

会议内容：

（1）总课题组工作汇报

武晓冬向各位专家和各指南课题组汇报第二批针灸临床实践指南总课题组的工作进程。

赵宏代表总课题组向各位专家和各指南课题组汇报临床指南的技术路线和目前临床指南课题组的工作进展。

（2）课题汇报及专家建议

各针灸临床实践指南小组向各位专家就指南的推荐方案和推荐意见进行了汇报。

与会专家在听取并审阅各课题组的推荐方案和推荐意见的基础上，就其存在的不足之处给予纠正和补充，并提出了自己的意见和建议。

（3）进度安排

各课题组的推荐方案和意见均已通过专家的讨论和修正。总课题组建议下一步工作安排：各临床指南课题组针对专家给出的意见就推荐方案进行进一步的修改和完善；针对各课题组提出的统一针灸临床专业术语和指南定稿格式的问题，总课题组经商议和明确后尽快给予回复；时间紧迫，要求各课题组在两周之内完成指南的最终定稿。

———————————